ORTHOPEDIC CLINICS OF NORTH AMERICA

www.orthopedic.theclinics.com

Nerve Injuries

April 2022 • Volume 53 • Number 2

Editor-in-Chief
FREDERICK M. AZAR

ELSEVIER

1600 John F. Kennedy Boulevard • Suite 1800 • Philadelphia, Pennsylvania, 19103-2899.

http://www.orthopedic.theclinics.com

ORTHOPEDIC CLINICS OF NORTH AMERICA Volume 53, Number 2
April 2022 ISSN 0030-5898, ISBN-13: 978-0-323-92008-7

Editor: Megan Ashdown
Developmental Editor: Ann Gielou Posedio

Orthopedic Clinics of North America (ISSN 0030-5898) is published quarterly by Elsevier Inc., 360 Park Avenue South, New York, NY 10010-1710. Months of issue are January, April, July, and October. Business and Editorial Offices: 1600 John F. Kennedy Blvd., Suite 1800, Philadelphia, PA 19103-2899. Customer Service Office: 3251 Riverport Lane, Maryland Heights, MO 63043. Periodicals postage paid at New York, NY and additional mailing offices. Subscription prices are $354.00 per year for (US individuals), $1,033.00 per year for (US institutions), $420.00 per year (Canadian individuals), $1,064.00 per year (Canadian institutions), $486.00 per year (international individuals), $1,064.00 per year (international institutions), $100.00 per year (US students), $100.00 per year for (Canadian students), $220.00 per year for (international students). Foreign air speed delivery is included in all *Clinics* subscription prices. All prices are subject to change without notice. **POSTMASTER:** Send change of address to *Orthopedic Clinics of North America*, **Elsevier Health Sciences Division, Subscription Customer Service, 3251 Riverport Lane, Maryland Heights, MO 63043. Customer Service (orders, claims, online, change of address):** Elsevier Health Sciences Division, Subscription Customer Service, **3251 Riverport Lane, Maryland Heights, MO 63043. Tel: 1-800-654-2452 (U.S. and Canada); 314-447-8871 (outside U.S. and Canada). Fax: 314-447-8029. E-mail:** journalscustomerservice-usa@elsevier.com **(for print support);** journalsonlinesupport-usa@elsevier.com **(for online support).**

Reprints. For copies of 100 or more, of articles in this publication, please contact the Commercial Reprints Department, Elsevier Inc., 360 Park Avenue South, New York, NY 10010-1710. Tel.: 212-633-3874; Fax: 212-633-3820; E-mail: reprints@elsevier.com.

Orthopedic Clinics of North America is covered in *MEDLINE/PubMed* (*Index Medicus*), *Cinahl, Excerpta Medica,* and *Cumulative Index to Nursing and Allied Health Literature.*

EDITORIAL BOARD

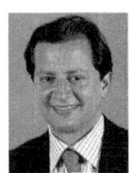
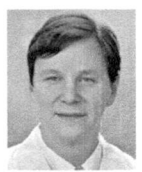
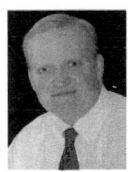
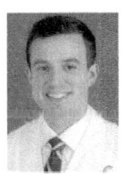
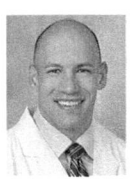
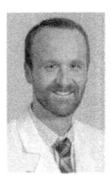

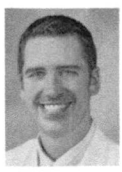
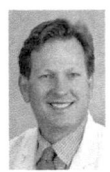
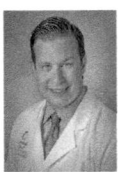
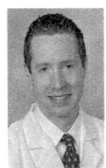
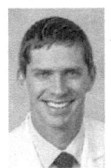
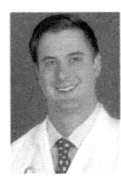

CONTRIBUTORS

EDITOR

FREDERICK M. AZAR, MD
Department of Orthopaedic Surgery and Biomedical Engineering, University of Tennessee-Campbell Clinic, Memphis, Tennessee, USA

AUTHORS

JOSEPH A. ABBOUD, MD
Professor, Department of Orthopaedic Surgery, Professor of Shoulder and Elbow Surgery, Rothman Orthopaedic Institute at Thomas Jefferson University, Philadelphia, Pennsylvania, USA

THOMAS R. ACOTT, MD
Faculty, The CORE Institute, Phoenix, Arizona, USA

DAVID BACKSTEIN, MD, MED, FRCSC
Associate Professor, University of Toronto, Head, Gluskin Granovsky Division of Orthopaedics, Mount Sinai Hospital, Medical Lead and Chair, Mount Sinai Centre for MSK Disease, Toronto, Ontario, Canada

MICHAEL D. BAIRD, MD
Department of Orthopaedic Surgery, Uniformed Services University-Walter Reed Department of Surgery, Walter Reed National Military Medical Center, Bethesda, Maryland, USA

ANDREW BOHM, PhD
Research Coordinator, Northwell Health— Lenox Hill Hospital, Department of Orthopaedics, New York, USA

LANDON BULLOCH, MD
Atrium Health Department of Orthopaedic Surgery, Charlotte, North Carolina, USA

ZACHARY BURNETT, MD
Resident Physician, Department of Orthopaedic Surgery, University of Virginia, Charlottesville, Virginia, USA

BLAS CATALANI, MD, MPH
Adjunct Professor, Department of Anesthesiology, The University of Tennessee Health Science Center, College of Medicine, UTROP/Regional One Health, Memphis, Tennessee, USA

DANIEL COHEN, MD
Adult Lower Extremity Reconstruction Unit, Mount Sinai Hospital, Gluskin Granovsky Division of Orthopaedics, University of Toronto, Toronto, Ontario, Canada

MOHAMMAD DAHER, BSc
Medical Student, Faculty of Medicine, Saint-Joseph University, Beirut, Lebanon

MICHAEL DALY, MD
Department of Orthopaedic Traumatology, University of Maryland, Baltimore, Maryland, USA

NISHANT DWIVEDI, MD
Resident Physician, Department of Orthopedic Surgery, Washington University in St. Louis, St Louis, Missouri, USA

CHRISTOPHER J. DY, MD, MPH
Associate Professor, Department of Orthopedic Surgery, Washington University in St. Louis, St Louis, Missouri, USA

DAVID A. FULLER, MD
Professor, Department of Orthopaedic Surgery, Cooper Medical School of Rowan University, Camden, New Jersey, USA

GRAHAM S. GOH, MD
Rothman Orthopaedic Institute at Thomas Jefferson University, Philadelphia, Pennsylvania, USA

RICHARD A. HILLESHEIM, MD
Department of Orthopaedic Surgery and
Biomedical Engineering, University of
Tennessee-Campbell Clinic, Memphis,
Tennessee, USA

HAYDEN S. HOLBROOK, MD
Department of Orthopaedic Surgery and
Biomedical Engineering, University of
Tennessee-Campbell Clinic, Memphis,
Tennessee, USA

JEFFREY E. JOHNSON, MD
Professor Emeritus, Department of
Orthopedic Surgery, Washington University in
St. Louis, St Louis, Missouri, USA

JERRY JONES, Jr, MD
Assistant Professor, Division Chief, Regional
Anesthesia and Acute Pain Management,
Department of Anesthesiology, The University
of Tennessee Health Science Center, College
of Medicine, UTROP/Regional One Health,
Memphis, Tennessee, USA

CHRIS LANGHAMMER, MD, PhD
Department of Orthopaedic Traumatology,
University of Maryland, Baltimore, Maryland,
USA

JAMES S. LIN, MD
Department of Orthopaedics, The Ohio State
University Wexner Medical Center, Columbus,
Ohio, USA

MICHAEL A. MONT, MD
Director of Clinical Trials, Northwell Health–
Lenox Hill Hospital, Department of
Orthopaedics, New York, New York, USA;
Orthopaedic Surgeon, Rubin Institute of
Advanced Orthopedics, Center for Joint
Preservation and Replacement, Sinai Hospital
of Baltimore, Baltimore, Maryland, USA

JAVAD PARVIZI, MD, FRCS
Rothman Orthopaedic Institute at Thomas
Jefferson University, Philadelphia,
Pennsylvania, USA

MANAN S. PATEL, MD
Resident Physician, Department of
Orthopaedic Surgery, Cooper University
Hospital, Camden, New Jersey, USA

AMBIKA E. PAULSON, MS
Medical Student, Georgetown University
School of Medicine, Washington, DC, USA

BENJAMIN K. POTTER, MD
Department of Orthopaedic Surgery,
Uniformed Services University-Walter Reed
Department of Surgery, Walter Reed National
Military Medical Center, Bethesda, Maryland,
USA

CHRISTOPHER H. RENNINGER, MD
Department of Orthopaedic Surgery,
Uniformed Services University-Walter Reed
Department of Surgery, Walter Reed
National Military Medical Center,
Bethesda, Maryland, USA; Department of
Orthopaedics, R Adams Cowley Shock
Trauma Center, University of Maryland
School of Medicine, Baltimore, Maryland,
USA

JOHN T. RICHARDS, MD
Department of Orthopaedic Surgery,
Uniformed Services University-Walter Reed
Department of Surgery, Walter Reed
National Military Medical Center,
Bethesda, Maryland, USA; Department of
Orthopaedics, R Adams Cowley Shock
Trauma Center, University of Maryland
School of Medicine, Baltimore, Maryland,
USA

JULIE BALCH SAMORA, MD, PhD
Department of Orthopaedics, Nationwide
Children's Hospital, The Ohio State University
Wexner Medical Center, Columbus, Ohio,
USA

GILES R. SCUDERI, MD
Donald and Barbara Zucker School of
Medicine at Hofstra/Northwell, Hempstead,
New York, USA; Vice-President Orthopaedic
Service Line, Northwell Health—Lenox Hill
Hospital, Department of Orthopaedics,
New York, New York, USA

JASON M. SOUZA, MD
Department of Plastic and Reconstructive
Surgery, The Ohio State University Wexner
Medical Center, Columbus, Ohio, USA

LEO SPECTOR, MD, MBA
Chief Quality Officer, OrthoCarolina Spine
Center, Charlotte, North Carolina,
USA

JOHN M. TARAZI, MD
Research Fellow, Department of
Orthopaedics, Northwell Health—Huntington

Hospital, Huntington, New York, USA; Donald and Barbara Zucker School of Medicine at Hofstra/Northwell, Hempstead, New York, USA

KIRK THOMPSON, MD
Campbell Clinic Orthopaedics, Memphis, Tennessee, USA

SCOTT M. TINTLE, MD
Department of Orthopaedic Surgery, Uniformed Services University-Walter Reed Department of Surgery, Walter Reed National Military Medical Center, Bethesda, Maryland, USA

WILLIAM J. WELLER, MD
Department of Orthopaedic Surgery and Biomedical Engineering, University of Tennessee-Campbell Clinic, Memphis, Tennessee, USA

BRIAN C. WERNER, MD
Associate Professor of Orthopaedic Surgery, University of Virginia, Charlottesville, Virginia, USA

THEOFANIS P. ZOIS, PA
Physician Assistant, Northwell Health—Lenox Hill Hospital, Department of Orthopaedics, New York, USA

CONTENTS

Preface   xv
Frederick M. Azar

Knee and Hip Reconstruction

Nerve Injuries in Total Knee Arthroplasty   123
Daniel Cohen and David Backstein

Nerve injury is one of the potential complications of total knee arthroplasty.
The extent of the injury includes motor and sensory dysfunction, either temporary or permanent. Although the consequences of nerve injury may be dramatic, the probability of occurrence during the course of primary knee
arthroplasty is low, around 0.12% to 0.4%. Local dressing removal and knee
flexion are imperative, and the initial investigations include ultrasound or MRI
and nerve conduction studies. The extent of recovery depends on the type
and severity of the initial nerve palsy; however, most patients are expected
to have at least a partial recovery.

Nerve Injuries Following Total Hip Arthroplasty: The Influence of Surgical   129
Approach
Graham S. Goh and Javad Parvizi

Nerve injuries following total hip arthroplasty are rare but devastating complications. The most important modifiable risk factor remains the choice of hip
approach and surgical technique applied. The risk of nerve injuries is related
to technical complexity of the procedure and anatomic variability of the
nerves. Surgeons should remain cognizant of inherent risk factors, variations
in the course and branching patterns of different nerves, and technical considerations of the surgical approach to mitigate risks. This article reviews the literature on postsurgical nerve injuries following total hip arthroplasty and
characterizes the influence of surgical approach on the risk of this
complication.

Elevated Pre-operative D-Dimer Levels Do Not Impact the Effect of Tranexamic   139
Acid on Revision Total Knee Arthroplasty
John M. Tarazi, Theofanis P. Zois, Andrew Bohm, Michael A. Mont, and
Giles R. Scuderi

The purpose of this study was to determine if elevated pre-operative D-dimer
levels in patients undergoing revision total knee arthroplasty (rTKA) pose an
increased risk of: (1) post-operative venous thromboemboli (VTE); (2) intraoperative blood loss; and (3) need for transfusion of blood products.
Eighty-nine patients who underwent rTKA by a single surgeon between
January 1, 2017, and December 31, 2019, met the inclusion criteria. Elevated
pre-operative D-dimer levels did not pose an increased risk of VTE, blood
loss, or transfusion of blood products, demonstrating that elevated pre-
operative D-dimer is not a contraindication to the use of tranexamic acid
for rTKA.

Trauma

Radial Nerve Injury in Humeral Shaft Fracture   **145**
Michael Daly and Chris Langhammer

> Radial nerve injury with humeral shaft fracture is common. Treatment options include expectant management, early exploration and repair, delayed reconstruction, nerve transfers, and tendon transfers. Knowledge of the appropriate application of these treatments will assist orthopedic surgeons and nerve surgeons in coordinating care for these patients.

Peripheral Nerve Management in Extremity Amputations   **155**
John T. Richards, Michael D. Baird, Scott M. Tintle, Jason M. Souza, Christopher H. Renninger, and Benjamin K. Potter

> The effective management of peripheral nerves in amputation surgery is critical to optimizing patient outcomes. Nerve-related pain after amputation is common, maybe a source of dissatisfaction and functional impairment, and should be considered in all amputees presenting with pain and dysfunction. While traction neurectomy or transposition has long been the standard of care, both regenerative peripheral nerve interface (RPNI) and targeted muscle reinnervation (TMR) have emerged as promising techniques to improve neuroma-related and phantom pain. A multi-disciplinary and multi-modal approach is essential for the optimal management of amputees both acutely and in the delayed or chronic setting.

Pediatrics

Brachial Plexus Birth Injuries   **167**
James S. Lin and Julie Balch Samora

> Brachial plexus birth injuries (BPBIs) are typically traction type injuries to the newborn that occur during the delivery process. Although the incidence of these injuries has overall decreased from 1.5 to around 0.9 per 1000 live births in the United States over the past 2 decades, these injuries remain common, with incidence holding fairly steady from 2008 to 2014. Shoulder dystocia is the strongest identified risk factor, imparting a 100-fold greater risk. The newborn's shoulder is caught behind the mother's pubic bone, and traction performed on the child during delivery results in injury to the brachial plexus. Other risk factors associated with BPBI include macrosomia (birthweight > 4.5 kg), heavy for gestational age infants, birth hypoxia, gestational diabetes, and forceps or vacuum-assisted delivery. Breech presentation has also been described as a risk factor in the past, but there have been more recent data that challenge this association.

Peripheral Nerve Block Complications in Children   **179**
Blas Catalani and Jerry Jones Jr

> Regional anesthesia, and in particular peripheral nerve block (PNB) techniques, complement existing anesthetic and pain management strategies and facilitate a comprehensively safer experience for the pediatric patient. Ultimately, the use of regional anesthesia cultivates a more satisfactory experience for all involved. Complication rates are very low, making PNBs a very safe option as proliferative incorporation of ultrasound technology has led to further enhancement of regional anesthesia safety and efficacy in the pediatric population.

Hand and Wrist

Digital Nerve Reconstruction   **187**
Thomas R. Acott

Tension-free primary digital nerve repair may be unachievable in the presence of a nerve defect and require digital nerve reconstruction. Multiple techniques are available for reconstruction of a digital nerve defect using conduits, autograft, and allograft. Multiple comparison studies exist in the literature, suggesting similar results with autograft and allograft reconstruction, with several comparison studies suggesting inferior outcomes with conduit repair.

Acute Carpal Tunnel Syndrome and Median Nerve Neurapraxia: A Review   **197**
Hayden S. Holbrook, Richard A. Hillesheim, and William J. Weller

Prompt diagnosis and treatment of acute injury to the median nerve after wrist trauma are paramount to a successful outcome. Neuropathy can occur primarily at the time of injury, secondary to unreduced fracture fragments or callus, or from prolonged immobilization in palmar flexion. Acute carpal tunnel syndrome is a surgical emergency that requires decompression. Progressively worsening pain and sensory disturbances in the median nerve distribution are findings that will distinguish an acute carpal tunnel syndrome from the less severe median nerve neurapraxia. This article describes the key differences between neurapraxia and acute compartment syndrome and their respective treatment.

Shoulder and Elbow

Incidence, Risk Factors, Prevention, and Management of Peripheral Nerve Injuries   **205**
Following Shoulder Arthroplasty
Manan S. Patel, Mohammad Daher, David A. Fuller, and Joseph A. Abboud

In this article, the authors review the incidence and causes of iatrogenic peripheral nerve injuries following shoulder arthroplasty and provide preventative measures to decrease nerve injury rate and management options. They describe common direct and indirect causes of injury such as laceration and retractor use versus arm positioning and lengthening, respectively. Preventative measures include an understanding of anatomy and high-risk locations in the shoulder, minimizing extreme ranges of arm motion and utilization of intraoperative nerve monitoring. Lastly, the authors review diagnosis and management of neurologic symptoms including how and when to use electrodiagnostic studies, nerve grafts, transfers, or muscle/tendon transfers.

Risk Factors, Management, and Prognosis of Brachial Plexopathy Following   **215**
Reverse Total Shoulder Arthroplasty
Zachary Burnett and Brian C. Werner

Brachial plexus injuries can have a significant impact on patient outcomes following RTSA by slowing the overall recovery and return of function. Risk factors for brachial plexopathy include traction injury related to arm positioning and exposure during the procedure, direct nerve injury from surgical dissection, and compression injury from retractor placement. Risk of nerve injury can be minimized by limiting the time spent with the arm extended and externally rotated and avoiding excessive traction on the arm during humeral preparation and implant insertion. Prompt identification of postoperative brachial plexopathy is important to optimize the recovery of function.

Foot and Ankle

Surgical Treatment of Foot Drop: Patient Evaluation and Peripheral Nerve Treatment Options   223
Nishant Dwivedi, Ambika E. Paulson, Jeffrey E. Johnson, and Christopher J. Dy

Foot drop is a common clinical condition which may substantially impact physical function and health-related quality of life. The etiologies of foot drop are diverse and a detailed history and physical examination are essential in understanding the underlying pathophysiology and capacity for spontaneous recovery. Patients presenting with acute foot drop or those without significant spontaneous recovery of motor deficits may be candidates for surgical intervention. The timing, mechanism, and severity of neural injury resulting in foot drop influence the selection of the most appropriate peripheral nerve surgery, which may include direct nerve repair, neurolysis, nerve grafting, or nerve transfer.

Surgical Treatment of Foot Drop: Pathophysiology and Tendon Transfers for Restoration of Motor Function   235
Nishant Dwivedi, Ambika E. Paulson, Christopher J. Dy, and Jeffrey E. Johnson

Foot drop is a common condition that may impact physical function and health-related quality of life. A detailed clinical history and physical examination are critical components of the initial evaluation of patients presenting with foot drop. Patients with refractory foot drop without spontaneous recovery of motor deficits, delayed presentation greater than 12 months from injury, or neural lesions that are not amenable to or have failed nerve reconstruction may be candidates for tendon transfers to restore active ankle dorsiflexion. The modified Bridle procedure is a dynamic tendon transfer that has demonstrated excellent functional outcomes in patients with refractory foot drop.

Spine Section

Cauda Equina Syndrome   247
Landon Bulloch, Kirk Thompson, and Leo Spector

Cauda equina syndrome (CES) involves compression of some or all of the lumbar and sacral peripheral nerve roots. However, there is a lack of consensus in the literature regarding the exact diagnosis criteria in this patient population. Much of the pathophysiology has been studied regarding the onset of this condition; however, the long-term effects are not able to be accurately predicted at this time. Recent literature has associated timing to surgical decompression, severity of symptoms at time of onset, and involvement of bladder dysfunction as prognostic indicators of CES.

NERVE INJURIES

FORTHCOMING ISSUES

July 2022
Soft Tissue Procedures
Michael J. Beebe, Clayton C. Bettin, Tyler J. Brolin, James H. Calandruccio, Christopher T. Cosgrove, Benjamin J. Grear, Benjamin M. Mauck, William M. Mihalko, Benjamin Sheffer, Kirk M. Thompson, and Patrick C. Toy, *Editors*

October 2022
Musculoskeletal Disorders
Michael J. Beebe, Clayton C. Bettin, Tyler J. Brolin, James H. Calandruccio, Christopher T. Cosgrove, Benjamin J. Grear, Benjamin M. Mauck, William M. Mihalko, Benjamin Sheffer, Kirk M. Thompson, and Patrick C. Toy, *Editors*

RECENT ISSUES

January 2022
Orthopedic Urgencies and Emergencies
Michael J. Beebe, Clayton C. Bettin, Tyler J. Brolin, James H. Calandruccio, Christopher T. Cosgrove, Benjamin J. Grear, Benjamin M. Mauck, William M. Mihalko, Benjamin Sheffer, Kirk M. Thompson, and Patrick C. Toy, *Editors*

October 2021
Fracture Care
Michael J. Beebe, Clayton C. Bettin, Tyler J. Brolin, James H. Calandruccio, Christopher T. Cosgrove, Benjamin J. Grear, Benjamin M. Mauck, William M. Mihalko, Benjamin Sheffer, David D. Spence, Kirk M. Thompson, and Patrick C. Toy, *Editors*

SERIES OF RELATED INTEREST

Foot and Ankle Clinics
https://www.foot.theclinics.com/
Clinics in Sports Medicine
https://www.sportsmed.theclinics.com/
Hand Clinics
https://www.hand.theclinics.com/
Physical Medicine and Rehabilitation Clinics
https://www.pmr.theclinics.com/

PREFACE

Damage to peripheral nerves can occur secondary to an accident or iatrogenic injury that compresses, stretches, or severs nerve fibers or secondary to a disease process, such as diabetes, rheumatoid arthritis, or even tumors. The symptoms of these injuries can be mild or severe, progressive or static. Regardless, treatment should be sought expeditiously to prevent permanent impairment. This issue mostly focuses on the treatment of peripheral nerve injuries related to trauma or surgical injury.

Dr David Cohen and Dr David Backstein describe nerve injury that can occur during primary knee replacement surgery, although this is quite rare. This injury, which includes motor and sensory dysfunction, can be temporary or permanent, depending on the type and severity. The authors emphasize immediate local dressing removal and knee flexion along with ultrasound or MRI and nerve conduction studies for prompt diagnosis. Drs Graham Goh and Javad Parvizi then discuss nerve injuries that can occur during total hip arthroplasty. Similar to the nerve palsy that can occur during knee arthroplasty, injury to the femoral cutaneous nerve can have devastating consequences. Their article presents a review of the literature, assessing the surgical techniques and their potential for nerve injury. Although not directly related to nerve injury in revision total knee arthroplasty, Dr Tarazi and colleagues set out to determine if elevated preoperative D-dimer levels pose an increased risk of venous thromboembolism, intraoperative blood loss, or need for transfusion and found that it does not increase the risk and is not a contraindication for using tranexamic acid.

Dr Michael Daley and Dr Chris Langhammer present an overview of radial nerve injury, which is a common occurrence in humeral shaft fractures. They discuss appropriate treatment options, such as early exploration and repair, delayed reconstruction, nerve transfers, and late tendon transfers. Dr John Richards and colleagues present management options for peripheral nerves in amputation surgery to minimize nerve-related pain and dysfunction. They note that in addition to traction neurectomy or transposition, regenerative peripheral nerve interface and targeted muscle reinnervation are promising new techniques to improve phantom pain and neuroma formation.

Brachial plexus injuries during birth remain fairly common in the United States. Although spontaneous recovery occurs in most patients, serial clinical examination is still necessary. Drs James Lin and Julie Samora review the indications for when early surgical intervention is necessary and present the most appropriate treatment options. Dr Blas Catalani and Dr Jerry Jones then describe peripheral nerve injuries that can result from nerve blocks in children. They emphasize that complication rates are very low, as incorporation of ultrasound technology has enhanced safety of regional nerve blocks in children.

Dr Acott provides an overview of techniques available for reconstruction of a digital nerve when tension-free primary repair is not possible. A review of the literature suggests similar results with autograft and allograft reconstruction, but inferior outcomes with conduit repair. Dr Hayden Holbrook and colleagues then present an in-depth review on acute carpal tunnel syndrome and median nerve neurapraxia. Distinguishing between these two is extremely important, as acute carpal tunnel syndrome is a surgical emergency.

Iatrogenic injury and brachial plexopathy are among the complications that can occur with shoulder arthroplasty. Dr Manan Patel and colleagues review the incidence and causes of iatrogenic peripheral nerve injuries in shoulder arthroplasty and offer preventative measures to decrease these complications. Dr Zach Burnett and Dr Brian Werner provide an overview of brachial plexopathy occurring with reverse total shoulder arthroplasty. These injuries can have a significant effect on outcomes and overall recovery. They recommend minimizing risk factors for injury, including avoiding excessive traction on the arm, taking care during exposure and surgical dissection, and limiting the time the arm is extended and externally rotated.

The surgical treatment of foot drop, a common clinical condition seen by foot and ankle specialists, is then discussed by Dr Nishant Dwivedi and colleagues. They describe the mechanism of injury and how this and the severity of injury will impact

Orthop Clin N Am 53 (2022) xv–xvi
https://doi.org/10.1016/j.ocl.2022.01.003
0030-5898/22/© 2022 Published by Elsevier Inc.

decisions on treatment, which may include neurolysis, nerve grafting or transfer, or direct repair. In a second article, the same authors present an overview of tendon transfer for restoration of motor function in foot drop.

Cauda equina syndrome is caused by compression of some or all of the lumbar and sacral peripheral nerve roots. Dr Landon Bulloch and colleagues reviewed the recent literature and found a lack of consensus regarding diagnostic criteria. They did find, however, that the time to surgical decompression, severity of symptoms at onset, and bladder dysfunction were prognostic indicators, although the long-term effects cannot be accurately predicted at this time.

We would like to thank the authors for their exceptional articles in this issue and hope readers will find these topics helpful in their practices.

Frederick M. Azar, MD
Department of Orthopaedic Surgery &
Biomedical Engineering
University of Tennessee–Campbell Clinic
1211 Union Avenue, Suite 510
Memphis, TN 38104, USA

E-mail address:
fazar@campbellclinic.com

Knee and Hip Reconstruction

Nerve Injuries in Total Knee Arthroplasty

Daniel Cohen, MD*, David Backstein, MD

KEYWORDS

- Nerve injury • Total knee • Arthroplasty • Common peroneal nerve

KEY POINTS

- The common peroneal and geniculate sensory nerves are at risk with knee arthroplasty.
- The incidence of nerve injury after TKA is generally believed to be in the range of 0.12% to 0.4%.
- Dysfunction of the common peroneal nerve may result in sensory impairment (lack of normal sensory to nerve, hypersensitivity and chronic pain) and/or motor dysfunction ("drop-foot").
- The extent of recovery depends on the type and severity of the initial nerve palsy, having most patients achieving some degree of recovery.
- Surgical nerve repair, including tendon transfers, is sometimes required.

BACKGROUND

Nerve injury is one of the potential complications of total knee arthroplasty (TKA). Generally speaking, neurologic injury may be temporary or permanent, can affect either or both motor and sensory branches and unlike most intraoperative complications, becomes apparent only after resolution of the operative anesthesia. Nerve injury can dramatically affect mobility and posture and is sometimes irreversible. This injury may be associated with pain, allodynia, neuroma formation, and cold sensitivity.[1,2] The risk of intraoperative complication is elevated in patients presenting with complex problems, such as the case of the multiply revised knee or one which requires correction of severe deformity. Primary TKA, however, is generally expected to result in high patient satisfaction and proceed in an uneventful manner for both patient and surgeon. Therefore, nerve injury, a devastating complication at any time, is even more dramatic in the context of primary TKA.

Although the consequences of nerve injury may be dramatic, the probability of occurrence during the course of primary knee arthroplasty is low. The incidence of nerve injury after TKA is generally believed to be in the range of 0.12% to 0.4%.[3,4] However, it should be noted that this incidence is based on large databases that included both primary and revision TKAs.

The following sections will review the anatomy of the nerves around the knee relevant to TKA, histopathology of nerve damage, incidence, treatment, and prognosis of neurologic injury.

NERVE ANATOMY AND POTENTIAL FOR INJURY

The nerves in the surgical zone of the knee, which are at greatest risk of injury during TKA, are the common peroneal nerve and the superficial sensory nerves around the skin incision (Fig. 1). The common peroneal nerve, one of the terminal branches of the sciatic nerve, has both motor and sensory functions. This nerve contains both the anterior tibial and peroneal nerves, which provide dorsiflexion and eversion power to the foot. It provides sensation to the lower lateral leg and dorsum of the foot. This nerve lies approximately 1.5 cm from the posterolateral tibial plateau and is interposed with the lateral gastrocnemius muscle at that

Adult Lower Extremity Reconstruction Unit, Mount Sinai Hospital, Gluskin Granovsky Division of Orthopaedics, University of Toronto, 600 University Avenue, #476D, Toronto, Ontario M5G 1X5, Canada
* Corresponding author.
E-mail address: donnycohen@gmail.com

Orthop Clin N Am 53 (2022) 123–127
https://doi.org/10.1016/j.ocl.2021.11.002

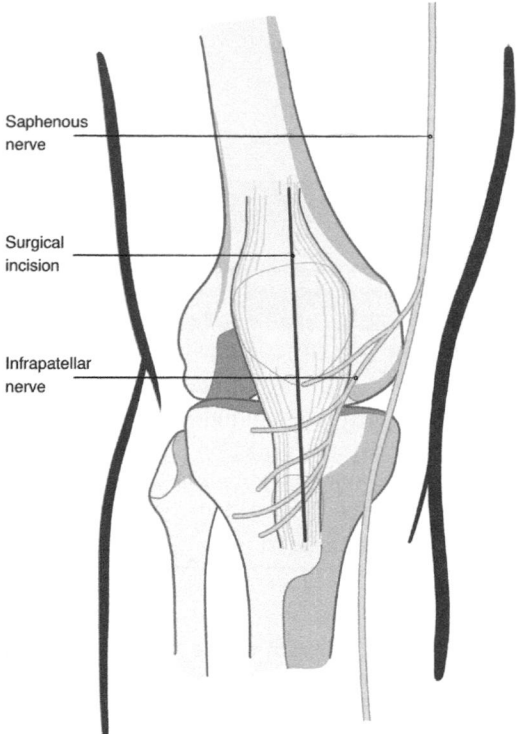

Saphenous
nerve

Surgical
incision

Infrapatellar
nerve

Fig. 1. Total knee arthroplasty incision crossing superficial sensory nerves.

level.[5] This provides relative protection of the nerve, although it is still at risk from stray surgical saw blades, and cautery. For example, the "pie-crust" technique, commonly used to release lateral soft tissue contractures in valgus knees, places the surgical blade near this nerve.

Both direct and indirect insults can injure the common peroneal nerve. Sources of direct insult include scalpel blades, cautery, saw blades, retractors, and other sharp instruments that may cause direct harm. Indirect injury may occur from forceful manipulation or elongation of the nerve, such as in the correction of severe valgus deformities.[3] In such deformity cases, the nerve and surrounding tissues are shortened because of the abnormal alignment anatomy. Correcting the alignment will elongate the course of the nerve, possibly causing a tension type of injury. Current understanding indicates that a maximal nerve elongation of 4% to 11% (up to 3 cm) can occur before nerve injury.[6]

The more common, generally unavoidable, nerve injury that occurs during the course of TKA relates to the superficial skin sensory nerves originating from the saphenous nerve. These nerves surround the knee from all sides and provide superficial sensation of the anterior knee. With the most common medial parapatellar

surgical approach, the incision itself divides these nerve fibers, and many patients describe a numb sensation around the surgical scar on either the medial or lateral side. It is possible for such nerve injuries to result in a neuroma formation, a possible etiology of postoperative pain. Much more common than the peroneal nerve insult, this deficit is sensory only, often transient, and generally has no impact on outcomes.

NERVE HISTOPATHOLOGY, DAMAGE AND REGENERATION

The peripheral nervous system is based on neurons, the primary cell, built of dendrites that receive information and axons which send it on. Some axons are wrapped with myelin covering to reduce the action potential dissipation. Myelinated and unmyelinated nerve fibers are bundled together in fascicles, covered with 3 layers of tissue—the endoneurium, perineurium, and epineurium. These layers provide structural support and protection to the neurons, and nerve injury classification is based on the injury to these specific layers.

Neuropraxia is the simplest form of nerve injury and is most likely to result in complete recovery. With this injury pattern, the nerve's myelin covering is damaged, hence the diminished signal. However, the actual nerve pathway is not harmed. Once the Schwann cells rebuild the myelin sheath, the nerve function should fully recover. This pattern is commonly found in chronic compression injuries.

The intermediate nerve injury level is axonotmesis. Here the actual nerve pathway, as opposed to the covering only, is damaged. The surrounding nerve sheath is still intact, but there is axonal discontinuity. Crush injuries exemplify this type of nerve damage. Wallerian degeneration occurs, and partial to full recovery can be expected.

Finally, neurotmesis occurs when the axon, myelin, and connective tissue components are damaged, disrupted, or transected, and is the most severe form of nerve injury. Recovery from neurotmesis requires surgical intervention, and the likelihood of full recovery is much lower. Transection of a nerve with a surgical saw blade or cautery would cause this devastating nerve insult.

NERVE REPAIR

During the recovery process from nerve injury, the damaged segment is first phagocytosed and degenerated, a process that takes up to several months.[7] In mild cases, the regenerative and repair processes begin almost immediately, but nerve regeneration will start only after the Wallerian degeneration has finished in more severe injuries. Sprouting of new axons by nerve fibers could take up to 6 weeks, reforming the nerve pathway. Depending on the extent of injury and defect size, axons may regenerate and begin to remyelinate at 6 to 8 weeks; however, the original thickness will never be achieved. On average, axonal growth occurs at a rate of 1 to 2 mm/d with a decreased rate in distal regions.[8] In severe injuries, prolonged denervation may lead to muscle atrophy. In the case of neurotmesis, surgical repair is imperative to restore the nerve infrastructure and align the correct nerve pathways for minimal scarring and adequate axonal recovery. Sometimes the use of nerve conduits or allografts is required.[9,10]

NERVE INJURY OUTCOME

Dysfunction of the common peroneal nerve may result in sensory impairment in the relevant anatomic distribution—ranging from lack of normal sensory to nerve hypersensitivity and chronic pain. Injury to the motor aspect could cause a "drop-foot"—the inability to dorsiflex the foot properly. Such an impairment may severely affect the patients' gait because raising the foot while walking is imperative. The severity of the insult (both functionally and visually) with the delayed recovery (sometimes irreversible damage) turns this nerve insult into one of the most significant potential surgical complications in knee arthroplasty. As mentioned earlier, the recovery is sometimes partial and may take months.

In contrast, injury to the geniculate sensory nerves around the surgical incision causes only local numbness around the incision and may recover within weeks to months.

INCIDENCE AND RECOVERY

The incidence of injury to the common peroneal nerve in knee arthroplasty is between 0.12% and 0.4%.[3,4] The combination of spinal conditions and valgus deformity holds the highest rate for postoperative nerve palsy.[3,11] Rheumatoid knees have also been associated with an elevated incidence of nerve injury.[12] The extent of recovery depends on the type and severity of the initial nerve palsy. At the 3.5-year mark, Schinsky and colleagues[12] found that 39% of patients with *complete* palsy had a full recovery, and 56% had partial recovery. In contrast, 66%

of patients with incomplete palsy recovered completely, and approximately 30% had an incomplete recovery. While awaiting recovery, treatment is supportive, initiating an ankle-foot orthosis to prevent falls.

The incidence of injury to the superficial skin sensory nerve is much higher (0.5%-53%) and occurrence is, to a large degree, inevitable.[13–15] There is no recommendation for specific treatment as the odds for sensation recovery are high, and the clinical implications are minimal.

PREVENTION

It is critical for all TKA surgeons to keep in mind the potential for nerve injury, particularly when performing complex surgery. Likewise, it is important for patients to fully understand the risks and implications of such an injury. In case of anatomic deformity, the surgeon must plan the maximal elongation that may be performed safely, at times necessitating under-correction of the alignment in the most severe cases. During the procedure, the surgeon and all assistants must be aware of the location of the peroneal nerve and prevent direct pressure and sharp contact. Owing to the necessity for anesthesia, there is currently no practical immediate marker informing dangerous closeness to the nerve. Several decades back, such neuromonitoring was suggested,[16] but as of today, no practical implication is in use.

EVALUATION AND TREATMENT

Patients should be assessed for nerve function as soon as the anesthetic effect allows. With any suspicion of nerve dysfunction, any dressing which might be causing local pressure should be removed, and the knee should be evaluated for a hematoma.[6] The leg should be positioned with the hip extended and knee flexed, to achieve maximal nerve relaxation.[6]

In the unfortunate case of peroneal nerve injury, the patient should be treated with an ankle-foot orthosis, holding the ankle in a neutral position, thus minimizing the risk of Achilles tendon shortening and improving posture. Anatomic evaluation of the nerve and surrounding anatomy to locate local structural compression and to assess nerve integrity should be performed by ultrasound or MRI.[17] A walking aid will often be needed for balance. Electromyography and nerve conduction studies should be performed for an objective assessment of the extent of the injury.[18]

Some authors have advocated for urgent surgical management in the scenario of direct damage to the common peroneal nerve, with relatively good results.[19] Others have found the surgical results to be suboptimal, with nerve recovery in about half the cases, depending on timing of intervention and extent of injury.[20,21] Combining nerve repair with tendon transfers achieves better outcomes. Posterior tibial tendon transfer to the dorsum of the foot has shown substantial improvement in functional outcomes.[22,23]

SUMMARY

When peroneal nerve injury occurs during elective TKA surgery, resulting in common peroneal palsy, it is a complication for both patient and surgeon. Prevention with all due precautions should be prioritized to prevent nerve injury from occurring. However, in the event of postoperative common peroneal nerve dysfunction, the patient should be treated immediately with local dressing decompression, knee flexion, and utilization of an ankle-foot orthosis. Nerve conduction studies and imaging are needed to further evaluate the extent of the injury. Spontaneous nerve recovery is generally expected in most cases and patient reassurance is imperative. Surgical intervention, sometimes combined with tendon transfers, may be indicated in cases of actual nerve fiber discontinuity, for better functional outcomes.

CLINICS CARE POINTS

- The common peroneal and geniculate sensory nerves are at risk with knee arthroplasty.
- The incidence of nerve injury after TKA is generally believed to be in the range of 0.12% to 0.4%.
- This common peroneal nerve, contains both the anterior tibial and peroneal nerves, which provide dorsiflexion and eversion power to the foot, and sensation to the lower lateral leg and dorsum of the foot.
- The nerve lies approximately 1.5 cm from the posterolateral tibial plateau and is interposed with the lateral gastrocnemius muscle at that level. This provides relative protection of the nerve, although it is still at risk from stray surgical saw blades, and cautery.

- Patients with abnormal alignment anatomy are at the highest risk for common peroneal nerve injury.
- Nerve injury to the superficial skin sensory nerves originating from the saphenous nerve is more common. The deficit is sensory only, often times transient, and generally has no impact on outcomes.
- With any suspicion of nerve dysfunction, any dressing which might be causing local pressure should be removed, and the leg should be positioned with the hip extended and knee flexed, to achieve maximal nerve relaxation.
- Immediate treatment includes:
  - Anatomic evaluation of the nerve and surrounding anatomy by ultrasound or MRI.
  - Walking aids.
  - Ankle orthosis.
  - Electromyography and nerve conduction studies.
  - Consider the need for immediate surgical intervention for nerve repair and tendon transfers.

DISCLOSURE

The authors have nothing to disclose.

REFERENCES

1. Dahlin LB. The role of timing in nerve reconstruction. Int Rev Neurobiol 2013;109:151–64.
2. James NF, Kumar AR, Wilke BK, et al. Incidence of encountering the infrapatellar nerve branch of the saphenous nerve during a midline approach for total knee arthroplasty. J Am Acad Orthop Surg Glob Res Rev 2019;3(12):e19, 00160.
3. Christ AB, Chiu YF, Joseph A, et al. Incidence and risk factors for peripheral nerve injury after 383,000 total knee arthroplasties using a New York State Database (SPARCS). J Arthroplasty 2019;34(10): 2473–8.
4. Carender CN, Bedard NA, An Q, et al. Common peroneal nerve injury and recovery after total knee arthroplasty: a systematic review. Arthroplast Today 2020;6(4):662–7.
5. Clarke HD, Schwartz JB, Math KR, et al. Anatomic risk of peroneal nerve injury with the "pie crust" technique for valgus release in total knee arthroplasty. J Arthroplasty 2004;19(1):40–4.
6. Nercessian OA, Ugwonali OF, Park S. Peroneal nerve palsy after total knee arthroplasty. J Arthroplasty 2005;20(8):1068–73.

7. Wineinger MA, Ellis WG. The clinical application of peripheral nerve pathology. Phys Med Rehabil Clin N Am 2001;12(2):237–51, vii.

8. Burnett MG, Zager EL. Pathophysiology of peripheral nerve injury: a brief review. Neurosurg Focus 2004;16(5):E1.

9. Boyd KU, Nimigan AS, Mackinnon SE. Nerve reconstruction in the hand and upper extremity. Clin Plast Surg 2011;38(4):643–60.

10. Siemionow M, Brzezicki G. Chapter 8: Current techniques and concepts in peripheral nerve repair. Int Rev Neurobiol 2009;87:141–72.

11. Shetty T, Nguyen JT, Sasaki M, et al. Risk factors for acute nerve injury after total knee arthroplasty. Muscle Nerve 2018;57(6):946–50.

12. Schinsky MF, Macaulay W, Parks ML, et al. Nerve injury after primary total knee arthroplasty. J Arthroplasty 2001;16(8):1048–54.

13. Jariwala AC, Parthasarathy A, Kiran M, et al. Numbness around the total knee arthroplasty surgical scar: prevalence and effect on functional outcome. J Arthroplasty 2017;32(7):2256–61.

14. Mistry D, O'Meeghan C. Fate of the infrapatellar branch of the saphenous nerve post total knee arthroplasty. ANZ J Surg 2005;75(9):822–4.

15. Lee SR, Dahlgren NJP, Staggers JR, et al. Cadaveric study of the infrapatellar branch of the saphenous nerve: Can damage be prevented in total knee arthroplasty? J Clin Orthop Trauma 2019; 10(2):274–7.

16. Unwin AJ, Thomas M. Intra-operative monitoring of the common peroneal nerve during total knee replacement. J R Soc Med 1994;87(11):701–3.

17. Girolami M, Galletti S, Montanari G, et al. Common peroneal nerve palsy due to hematoma at the fibular neck. J Knee Surg 2013;26(Suppl 1): S132–5.

18. Zywiel MG, Mont MA, McGrath MS, et al. Peroneal nerve dysfunction after total knee arthroplasty: characterization and treatment. J Arthroplasty 2011;26(3):379–85.

19. Garozzo D, Ferraresi S, Buffatti P. Surgical treatment of common peroneal nerve injuries: indications and results. A series of 62 cases. J Neurosurg Sci 2004;48(3):105–12 [discussion: 112].

20. Giuseffi SA, Bishop AT, Shin AY, et al. Surgical treatment of peroneal nerve palsy after knee dislocation. Knee Surg Sports Traumatol Arthrosc 2010; 18(11):1583–6.

21. George SC, Boyce DE. An evidence-based structured review to assess the results of common peroneal nerve repair. Plast Reconstr Surg 2014;134(2): 302e–11e.

22. Park JS, Casale MJ. Posterior tibial tendon transfer for common peroneal nerve injury. Clin Sports Med 2020;39(4):819–28.

23. Yeap JS, Birch R, Singh D. Long-term results of tibialis posterior tendon transfer for drop-foot. Int Orthop 2001;25(2):114–8.

Nerve Injuries Following Total Hip Arthroplasty

The Influence of Surgical Approach

Graham S. Goh, MD, Javad Parvizi, MD, FRCS*

KEYWORDS

- Hip arthroplasty • Complication • Approach • Direct anterior • Nerve palsy • Nerve injury

---

KEY POINTS

- Nerve injury during total hip arthroplasty (THA) is an uncommon but potentially devastating complication.
- The optimal surgical approach in THA has resurfaced as a topic of debate within the arthroplasty community recently.
- Despite the oft-cited benefits of the direct anterior approach (DA), a higher incidence of lateral femoral cutaneous nerve and femoral nerve palsies has been reported with this approach.
- This article reviews the literature on nerve injuries after THA and characterizes the influence of surgical approach on the risk of this complication.

INTRODUCTION

Total hip arthroplasty (THA) is one of the most successful surgical procedures.[1] Despite its proven efficacy, peripheral nerve palsy is an uncommon but potentially devastating complication that can occur following THA. The incidence of nerve injury has been estimated to be 0.17% to 3.3% after primary THA,[2–11] which may increase to 7.6% after revision THA.[2,5,6] Neurologic injuries not only hinder the functional recovery of THA patients, but also result in delayed return to work and long-term functional deficits if they do not resolve.[3,10,12] Of note, patients with nerve palsies lasting for 2 or more years after surgery have a lower likelihood of regaining neurologic function.[13] It is thus not surprising that postsurgical nerve injury has been shown to be the most common reason for medical malpractice litigation following THA in the United States.[14,15] Consequently, a better understanding of the factors influencing the risk of nerve injury is paramount.[16] Although it is often difficult to determine a cause in most cases, common causes of nerve palsies include

compression from retraction or hematoma formation, contusion, traction, iatrogenic laceration, vascular compromise, or thermal injury from cement.[2,5–8,10,11,17,18] Patient factors, such as female gender, hip dysplasia, and posttraumatic arthritis, and operative factors including revision procedures, cementless fixation, and aggressive anticoagulation, have also been shown to increase the risk of nerve palsies in THA.[2,10,11,19]

The optimal surgical approach in THA has recently resurfaced as a topic of debate within the arthroplasty community. Because of the growing trend toward outpatient joint replacement,[20] the direct anterior (DA) approach has gained attention as a muscle-sparing approach that minimizes blood loss and soft tissue trauma, enhances postoperative recovery, and reduces dislocation risk following THA.[21] However, a higher rate of lateral femoral cutaneous nerve (LFCN) and femoral nerve palsies could attenuate the clinical benefits gained from this approach.[22–24] One recent meta-analysis further suggested that the risk of nerve palsy was lowest

---

Rothman Orthopaedic Institute at Thomas Jefferson University, Philadelphia, PA, USA

* Corresponding author. Rothman Orthopaedic Institute, 125 South 9th Street, Suite 1000, Philadelphia, PA 19107.

E-mail address: javad.parvizi@gmail.com

Orthop Clin N Am 53 (2022) 129–137
https://doi.org/10.1016/j.ocl.2021.12.002

with the posterolateral approach, although a high degree of heterogeneity was observed in the pooled data.[25] In view of the rarity of postsurgical nerve injuries, speculation on the association between different THA approaches and the risk of various peripheral nerve injuries has been largely based on anatomic relations, and no evidence-based consensus has been reached regarding the optimal surgical approach to minimize this complication.

This article reviews the literature on postsurgical nerve injuries following THA and characterizes the influence of surgical approach on the risk of this complication.

SCIATIC NERVE

The most frequently injured nerve during THA is the sciatic nerve.[5] The incidence of this complication is 1.5% after primary THA and 3% to 8% in the revision setting.[5,7] The sciatic nerve arises from the L4-S3 nerve roots of the lumbar plexus. It exits the pelvis through the greater sciatic foramen, typically below piriformis,[26] although this relationship has been shown to vary greatly.[27,28] The type A variant, wherein the nerve exits below the piriformis as a single bundle, is most commonly encountered (85%). Five other variations where the sciatic nerve divides before exiting the pelvis have also been described.[28] The sciatic nerve descends in the posterior compartment of the thigh, deep to the biceps femoris and superficial to the adductor magnus, before entering the popliteal fossa. Sciatic nerve injuries usually affect the peroneal division,[29] presenting with weak dorsiflexion of the ankle and foot drop, or even complete paralysis of all the foot and ankle muscles in severe cases. Sensory disturbances, such as radiating buttock and leg pain or numbness, may also occur. Clinical findings may manifest within a month or up to 2 years following THA.[30]

The risk of sciatic nerve injury is highest with the posterior approach, and has been reported to occur in 0.6% of THA cases.[3] Although approximately 50% of patients have an unknown cause for the nerve injury,[31,32] some studies have attributed this to compression of the sciatic nerve between the ischium and gluteus maximus tendon.[33] Edwards and colleagues[6] analyzed 10 patients with sciatic nerve injuries and observed that limb-lengthening exceeded 4 cm in four cases. Malpositioning of a retractor is also an important cause of iatrogenic sciatic nerve damage.[24,31,34] At its posterior location in relationship to the greater trochanter, the sciatic nerve may be compressed by the trochanteric

retractor when retracting the femur posteriorly to expose the acetabulum.[35] Based on MRI of 263 hips, Wang and colleagues[36] found that the mean distance of the sciatic nerve from the posterior rim of the acetabulum was 1.96 cm and 1.94 cm in normal and dysplastic hips, respectively. A reduced distance was associated with female gender and smaller stature. Excessive manipulation of the lower extremity may also predispose to sciatic nerve injury. This may occur during preparation of the femoral canal and trialing of implants during THA. Overzealous traction, external rotation, or extension during a DA THA may lead to a stretch injury and sciatic nerve palsy.[37] As the peroneal nerve wraps around the fibular head, the peroneal division is at an increased risk of tethering and traction injury.[38] Moreover, the peroneal nerve has sparse connective tissue and larger funiculi, limiting its capacity to elongate.[31,33] Avoiding excessive traction during limb extension may help to mitigate this risk. Another possible cause is nerve ischemia. Sunderland[39] reported that the inferior gluteal artery, medial femoral circumflex artery, and perforating arteries of the profunda femoris supplied the sciatic nerve. Consequently, dissection of the short external rotators and mobilization of the nerve during a posterior approach could lead to vascular compromise. Direct laceration of the nerve could also occur if the posterior femoral cortex is breached during reaming. Other established modifiable risk factors include tobacco use and aggressive anticoagulation after THA,[6,40] whereas unmodifiable risk factors, such as preexisting spinal disease, hip dysplasia, and age older than 50 years have been suggested.[5,18] Surgeons should be cognizant of these risk factors when counseling patients regarding the risk of nerve injury after THA.

FEMORAL NERVE

The femoral nerve is derived from L2-L4 of the lumbar plexus, descending within the psoas muscle and passing deep to the inguinal ligament to reach the lateral aspect of the femoral triangle. It then splits into terminal motor branches to supply the muscles in the anterior thigh. The femoral nerve also receives sensory input from the hip and knee joints, and the anteromedial thigh before it becomes the saphenous nerve.[41] Femoral nerve palsies present with varying deficits in knee extension because of quadriceps weakness (ranging from subtle knee buckling to complete motor paralysis[42]) and sensory disturbances in the anteromedial thigh and medial leg.[22] Motor impairment from femoral nerve palsy may result in difficulty ambulating and has been associated with an increased risk of falls.[43]

The incidence of femoral nerve injury in THA has been reported to be 0.01% to 2.4%,[11,13,17,22] and 0% to 5% for DA THA in particular.[22,37] Compared with other approaches, the incidence of this complication was found to be 15 times higher in patients undergoing THA through a DA (0.40%) or anterolateral (0.64%) approach.[22] Because of its proximity to the anterior acetabular wall, positioning of the anterior retractors when exposing the acetabulum can lead to femoral nerve injury.[9,44] This is an important consideration, especially with the DA approach.[44,45] The mean distance between the femoral nerve and anterior acetabular rim has been shown to range between 1.8 and 2.2 cm.[46] A recent study by Yoshino and colleagues[47] dissected 84 cadaveric hips and found that the mean minimum distances from the femoral nerve were 33.2 mm, 24.4 mm, 18.4 mm, 16.6 mm, 17.9 mm, and 23.2 mm at 0°, 30°, 60°, 90°, 120°, and 150°, respectively, with 0° being defined as the intersection point on the acetabular rim for a line drawn between the anterior inferior iliac spine and center of the hip. Importantly, the distance was shortest at 90°, placing the nerve at the greatest risk during anterior retractor placement. Another cadaveric study using computed tomography scans demonstrated that retractor placement at the region of the anterior inferior iliac spine was furthest from the neurovascular bundle.[34] Similarly, Sullivan and colleagues[48] found that placing the anterior retractor superiorly helped to mitigate the risk of femoral nerve injury in DA THA. Consistent with these findings, Ishimatsu and colleagues[44] performed intraoperative neuromonitoring and noted that moving the retractors inferiorly along the acetabular rim brought it into closer proximity to the femoral nerve. In addition to direct compression from retractor placement,[46] indirect compression can occur from retraction of the iliopsoas.[49] Large osteophytes on the anterior acetabulum may result in poor contact between the retractor and the bony rim, increasing the risk of slippage and resultant nerve injury.[42,45] Another common cause is femoral nerve stretching from excessive limb-lengthening, a finding that has also been reported in studies on nonanterior approaches.[2,5,10,50] Additionally, hyperextension, extension, and adduction maneuvers during broaching and trialing may predispose to femoral nerve injury,[48] although this may be avoided by reducing traction on the limb. Thermal injury, iatrogenic laceration, and compression of nerve by hematoma from aggressive anticoagulation are other known causes of femoral nerve injury.[13,22]

SUPERIOR GLUTEAL NERVE

The superior gluteal nerve originates from L4-S1 of the lumbar plexus, passing above the piriformis when exiting the greater sciatic foramen before dividing into superior and inferior branches.[43,51] Two anatomic variants of the division have been described: the spray and transverse neural trunk variants.[52] The superior gluteal nerve innervates the gluteus medius and minimus and the tensor fasciae lata (TFL).[53] Injury can result in paralysis of these muscles, causing weak abduction and a Trendelenburg gait.[51] Notwithstanding, injury to the terminal branches supplying the TFL can go undiagnosed, because some patients may remain asymptomatic without functional impairment or cosmetic issues,[51] albeit others may experience atrophy and fatty infiltration of the TFL.[54,55]

The association between superior gluteal nerve injury and the Hardinge and Watson-Jones approaches have been well described.[51,56,57] This may occur especially if the gluteus medius is dissected 5 cm proximal to the greater trochanter during the direct lateral or anterolateral approach.[53,58] Unis and colleagues[56] analyzed MRI scans of patients undergoing THA using an anterolateral approach and noted fatty infiltration of the TFL in 42% of patients at a median of 9.4 months. More recently, the risk of superior gluteal nerve injury has also been demonstrated in DA THA.[51] One cadaveric study of 15 hips found that the distance between the superior gluteal nerve and the top of the greater trochanter was 3.9 cm as it crossed the interval between the TFL and gluteus medius.[55] This is an important consideration when excessively retracting the TFL during femoral broaching, because the terminal branches of the inferior division passes through the proximal half of the muscle.[51,55] Intracapsular retractor placement has been suggested to minimize nerve injury.[59] In a separate cadaveric study by Grob and colleagues[51] on 19 specimens, the entry point of the nerve was noted to be within 10 mm of the entry point of the ascending branch of the lateral circumflex femoral artery, prompting them to conclude that the artery could be used as an anatomic landmark to avoid damage of the terminal branches. Clamping, coagulation, or ligation of this artery close to the TFL may result in damage to these branches and TFL atrophy.[51] Superior gluteal nerve injury can also occur when incorrectly extending the DA approach proximally.[51,60]

When comparing the degree of damage to the TFL following a minimally invasive anterior and posterior approach, Meneghini and colleagues[60] reported that all cadaveric specimens in the DA group had damage to the TFL, with the midsubstance of TFL (at the entry point of the superior gluteal nerve) being the most common site of damage. Corroborating these findings, Takada and colleagues[54] analyzed computed tomography scans of 30 patients and found that the cross-sectional area of the TFL was significantly lower following DA THA compared with anterolateral THA, and MRI showed greater fatty infiltration of the muscle in the former group, although there was ultimately no significant difference in clinical outcomes. Fatty atrophy of the TFL was again demonstrated in an MRI study by Kawasaki and colleagues[61] following DA THA. Although direct TFL injury from broaching or retraction may account for these findings, it is also possible that subtle injury to the terminal branches may contribute to these TFL changes.

LATERAL FEMORAL CUTANEOUS NERVE

The LFCN is a sensory nerve that originates from L2 and L3 of the lumbar plexus. The nerve exits at the lateral border of the psoas, traversing across the iliacus and reaching the inferior aspect of the anterior superior iliac spine.[62] Four variations in branching have been described (classical, late, primary femoral, and trifurcate).[62,63] Branches of the LFCN often pass through the surgical interval between the TFL and sartorius,[62] piercing the belly of the TFL and supplying the anterolateral skin of the thigh.[64] Although nerve injury may not result in major functional impairment,[41,65] injury to the LFCN can cause symptoms of numbness or dysesthesia in the affected region,[45] with the former symptom being more prevalent and the latter having a greater impact on quality of life.[62,66]

Existing literature has demonstrated a highly variable incidence of LFCN injury following DA THA (0.1%–81%).[41,54,62,64,67–70] Rudin and colleagues[62] hypothesized that the anatomic branching pattern of the LFCN in the proximal thigh and the surgical technique during the DA approach could influence the risk of LFCN injury, although they qualified that a certain degree of injury may be inevitable in a third of patients.

Studies have shown that blunt dissection in the surgical interval of the TFL and sartorius may increase the risk of LFCN injury in DA THA.[62,69,70] This was supported by Takada and colleagues,[54] who observed a 23% rate of injury on the DA side versus 0% on the anterolateral side, despite a near-identical skin incision made in both approaches. Ozaki and colleagues[71] also suggested that a smaller femoral offset and smaller long axis of the TFL were associated with an increased risk of LFCN neuropraxia after DA THA. Although a more lateral incision has been proposed to minimize the risk of LFCN injury, Bartlett and colleagues[63] encountered the LFCN in nearly half of their cohort even when a 2-cm lateralization was made. The different branching patterns of the nerve may be a bigger risk factor for nerve injury, because the late branching pattern has been shown to increase the risk of damage because of the perpendicular orientation of the nerve in relationship to the surgical incision. Although it is difficult to predict the anatomy of the nerve before surgery, surgeons should have knowledge of the different anatomic variations to minimize the risk of iatrogenic injury when the branches are encountered intraoperatively.

OTHER NERVES

The pudendal and obturator nerves are less commonly injured during THA. The pudendal nerve arises from S2-S4 and travels posterior to the sacrospinous ligament and medial to the ischial spine. The nerve passes between the sacrotuberous and sacrospinal ligaments before entering the pudendal canal.[72] Nerve deficits may manifest as sensory disturbances in the perineum and sexual dysfunction.[73,74] Excessive stretching or direct compression against an inadequately padded perineal post during limb traction are causes of nerve injury following DA THA.[73]

Obturator nerve injury may also rarely occur in THA.[18,31] The nerve arises from L2-4 of the lumbar plexus, passing through the psoas muscle, traveling medially over the pelvic brim, and exiting via the obturator foramen. An injury to the nerve may result in sensory deficits along the medial thigh and weakness of the adductor muscles. A case series by Siliski and Scott[75] found that cement extrusion in THA could lead to obturator nerve injury. In a large cohort study of 2012 hip replacements, only one procedure was complicated by obturator nerve injury, which was again attributed to cement extrusion.[7] Because cemented acetabular components are no longer used, the incidence of this complication is likely even lower in contemporary practice. Disruption of the acetabular floor or anterior wall may also predispose to obturator nerve injury.[76]

DIAGNOSIS

Because the clinical manifestations of nerve palsies following THA may be subtle, additional investigations, such as electromyography (EMG) or nerve conduction studies, may be necessary to confirm the diagnosis. Studies have shown that clinical examination alone may underdiagnose postsurgical nerve injuries.[7,9] In contrast, EMG studies have shown that the incidence of subclinical nerve injuries may reach up to 70% after THA.[8] A handheld dynamometer can also be used to objectively measure muscle strength, and measurements from the contralateral limb may serve as a reference to ascertain decreased motor function in the affected leg.[22]

PROGNOSIS

The recovery potential and duration of various nerve palsies may vary among the different nerves. Some authors have suggested that most postoperative nerve injuries never fully recover, regardless of whether they were incomplete or complete injuries.[10,77] Nercessian and colleagues[77] found that nerve injuries in 27% of primary cases and 43% of revision cases were permanent. However, femoral nerve injuries, in general, have a more favorable prognosis and predictable recovery compared with that of sciatic nerve injuries.[5,32] Siguier and colleagues[78] found that both cases of femoral nerve injury in DA THA showed complete recovery within the first postoperative year. This finding was echoed by Hoshino and colleagues,[42] who also noted electrophysiologic signs of recovery within weeks after surgery. Another study reported complete recovery of femoral nerve palsies within 6 months.[79] Regarding sciatic nerve injuries, Clawson and Seddon[80] noted differences in recovery potential between the tibial and peroneal divisions, with full return of function in 79% and 36% of cases, respectively. Notwithstanding, few studies have evaluated the long-term prognosis of postsurgical nerve injuries, taking account the extent of injury and the specific nerve palsy.[31,81] Zappe and colleagues[82] analyzed 2225 primary and revision THAs, and stratified femoral, sciatic, and superior gluteal nerve palsies based on muscle power (severe, 0–2; light 3–4) using EMG. The authors found

that 34 patients (1.5%) had nerve injuries, 17 (50%) of which regained their function completely after 2 years, with no difference in recovery potential among the three nerves. LFCN injuries may result in permanent sensory deficits, although patients are nonetheless able to accommodate these symptoms with time. Based on current evidence, it is clear that recovery following postsurgical nerve injuries may be highly variable,[16] and further research is needed to elucidate the long-term outcomes of patients that suffer these rare complications.

SUMMARY

Nerve injuries following THA are rare but devastating complications. The interest in this topic comes amid the growing popularity of the DA approach, which has been shown to yield a 2.8% incidence of clinically significant nerve damage after surgery.[83] Although multiple risk factors, such as hip dysplasia and prior hip surgery, are well described, the most important modifiable risk factor remains the choice of hip approach and surgical technique applied. Some authors have suggested that surgeon experience and learning curve could result in an increased rate of complications[84,85] and nerve injury in particular,[2] whereas others have questioned this relationship.[42] Nonetheless, the risk of nerve injuries seems to be closely related to the technical complexity of the procedure and anatomic variability of the nerves. Surgeons should remain cognizant of inherent risk factors, variations in the course and branching patterns of different nerves, and technical considerations of the surgical approach (eg, retractor placement) to mitigate these risks.

CLINICS CARE POINTS

- Nerve injury following total hip arthroplasty (THA) is a rare but devastating complication. The most important modifiable risk factor remains the choice of hip approach and surgical technique applied.

- In addition to excessive limb-lengthening and overzealous traction, malpositioning of retractors during any surgical approach is an important avoidable cause of iatrogenic nerve damage.

- Sciatic nerve injury is most common with the posterior approach. At its posterior location in relationship to the greater trochanter, the sciatic nerve may be compressed by the trochanteric retractor when retracting the femur posteriorly to expose the acetabulum. The mean distance of the sciatic nerve from the posterior rim of the acetabulum is 1.96 cm and 1.94 cm in normal and dysplastic hips, respectively. Of note, this distance may be reduced in patients who are female and smaller in stature.

- Femoral nerve injury is most common with the direct anterior (DA) approach. Positioning of the anterior retractors when exposing the acetabulum can lead to femoral nerve injury. The mean distance between the femoral nerve and anterior acetabular rim has been shown to range between 1.8 and 2.2 cm. The distance is shortest at 90° (with 0° being defined as the intersection point on the acetabular rim for a line drawn between the anterior inferior iliac spine and center of the hip).

- Superior gluteal nerve injury is more common with the direct lateral and anterolateral approaches. However, the risk of superior gluteal nerve injury has also been recently demonstrated in DA THA. This can occur with excessive retraction of the tensor fasciae lata (TFL) during femoral broaching, as the terminal branches of the inferior division of this nerve pass through the proximal half of the muscle. The ascending branch of the lateral circumflex femoral artery can be used as an anatomic landmark to avoid damage of these branches.

DISCLOSURE

Neither author has anything to disclose in relation to this review, and no funding was received.

REFERENCES

1. Learmonth ID, Young C, Rorabeck C. The operation of the century: total hip replacement. Lancet 2007;370:1508–19.
2. Johanson NA, Pellicci PM, Tsairis P, et al. Nerve injury in total hip arthroplasty. Clin Orthop 1983;214–22.
3. Navarro RA, Schmalzried P, Amstutz HC. Surgical approach and nerve palsy in total hip arthroplasty. J Arthroplasty 1995;10:1–5.
4. Wasielewski RC, Crossett LS, Rubash HE. Neural and vascular injury in total hip arthroplasty. Orthop Clin North Am 1992;23:219–35.
5. Schmalzried TP, Amstutz HC, Dorey FJ. Nerve palsy associated with total hip replacement. Risk factors and prognosis. J Bone Jt Surg 1991;73:1074–80.
6. Edwards BN, Tullos HS, Noble PC. Contributory factors and etiology of sciatic nerve palsy in total hip arthroplasty. Clin Orthop 1987;218:136–41.
7. Weber ER, Daube JR, Coventry MB. Peripheral neuropathies associated with total hip arthroplasty. J Bone Jt Surg 1976;58:66–9.
8. Solheim LF, Hagen R. Femoral and sciatic neuropathies after total hip arthroplasty. Acta Orthop Scand 1980;51:531–4.
9. Weale AE, Newman P, Ferguson IT, et al. Nerve injury after posterior and direct lateral approaches for hip replacement. A clinical and electrophysiological study. J Bone Joint Surg Br 1996;78:899–902.
10. Farrell CM, Springer BD, Haidukewych GJ, et al. Motor nerve palsy following primary total hip arthroplasty. J Bone Jt Surg-am 2005;87-A:2619–25.
11. Brown GD, Swanson EA, Nercessian OA. Neurologic injuries after total hip arthroplasty. Am J Orthop Belle Mead NJ 2008;37:191–7.
12. Oldenburg M, Müller RT. The frequency, prognosis and significance of nerve injuries in total hip arthroplasty. Int Orthop 1997;21:1–3.
13. Fox AJS, Bedi A, Wanivenhaus F, et al. Femoral neuropathy following total hip arthroplasty: review and management guidelines. Acta Orthop Belg 2012;78:145–51.
14. Samuel LT, Sultan AA, Rabin JM, et al. Medical malpractice litigation following primary total joint arthroplasty: a comprehensive, nationwide analysis of the past decade. J Arthroplasty 2019;34:S102–7.
15. Bokshan SL, Ruttiman RJ, DePasse JM, et al. Reported litigation associated with primary hip and knee arthroplasty. J Arthroplasty 2017;32:3573–7.e1.
16. Hasija R, Kelly JJ, Shah NV, et al. Nerve injuries associated with total hip arthroplasty. J Clin Orthop Trauma 2018;9:81–6.
17. Simmons C, Izant TH, Rothman RH, et al. Femoral neuropathy following total hip arthroplasty. Anatomic study, case reports, and literature review. J Arthroplasty 1991;6(Suppl):S57–66.
18. Yang I-H. Neurovascular injury in hip arthroplasty. Hip Pelvis 2014;26:74.
19. Christ AB, Chiu Y, Joseph A, et al. Risk factors for peripheral nerve injury after 207,000 total hip arthroplasties using a New York State Database (Statewide Planning and Research Cooperative System). J Arthroplasty 2019;34:1787–92.
20. Rozell JC, Ast MP, Jiranek WA, et al. Outpatient Total Joint Arthroplasty: The New Reality. J Arthroplasty 2021;36(7S):S33–9.
21. Flevas DA, Tsantes AG, Mavrogenis AF. Direct anterior approach total hip arthroplasty Revisited. JBJS Rev 2020;8:e0144.
22. Fleischman AN, Rothman RH, Parvizi J. Femoral nerve palsy following total hip arthroplasty: incidence and course of recovery. J Arthroplasty 2018;33:1194–9.
23. Dahm F, Aichmair A, Dominkus M, et al. Incidence of lateral femoral cutaneous nerve lesions after

direct anterior approach primary total hip arthroplasty: a literature review. Orthop Traumatol Surg Res 2021;102956. https://doi.org/10.1016/j.otsr.2021.102956.

24. Vajapey SP, Morris J, Lynch D, et al. Nerve injuries with the direct anterior approach to total hip arthroplasty. JBJS Rev 2020;8:e0109.

25. Migliorini F, Trivellas A, Eschweiler J, et al. Nerve palsy, dislocation and revision rate among the approaches for total hip arthroplasty: a Bayesian network meta-analysis. Musculoskelet Surg 2021;105:1–15.

26. McMinn RM, Hutchings RT, Pegington J, et al. A colour atlas of human anatomy. Year Book Medical Publishers; 1988.

27. Beaton LE, Anson BJ. The relation of the sciatic nerve and of its subdivisions to the piriformis muscle. Anat Rec 1937;70:1–5.

28. Tomaszewski KA, Graves MJ, Henry BM, et al. Surgical anatomy of the sciatic nerve: a meta-analysis. J Orthop Res Off Publ Orthop Res Soc 2016;34:1820–7.

29. De Fine M, Romagnoli M, Zaffagnini S, et al. Sciatic Nerve Palsy following Total Hip Replacement: Are Patients Personal Characteristics More Important than Limb Lengthening? A Systematic Review. Biomed Res Int 2017.

30. Xu LW, Veeravagu A, Azad TD, et al. Delayed presentation of sciatic nerve injury after total hip arthroplasty: neurosurgical considerations, diagnosis, and management. J Neurol Surg Rep 2016;77:e134–8.

31. DeHart MM, Riley LH. Nerve injuries in total hip arthroplasty. J Am Acad Orthop Surg 1999;7:101–11.

32. Della Valle CJ, Di Cesare PE. Complications of total hip arthroplasty: neurovascular injury, leg-length discrepancy, and instability. Bull NYU Hosp Jt Dis 2002;60:134.

33. Hurd JL, Potter HG, Dua V, et al. Sciatic nerve palsy after primary total hip arthroplasty: a new perspective. J Arthroplasty 2006;21:796–802.

34. Shubert D, Madoff S, Milillo R, et al. Neurovascular structure proximity to acetabular retractors in total hip arthroplasty. J Arthroplasty 2015;30:145–8.

35. Koch S, Tillmann B. Anatomical comment: Hohmann retractor. A source of danger to the sciatic nerve. Oper Orthopadie Traumatol 1997;9:27–33.

36. Wang T-I, Chen H-Y, Tsai C-H, et al. Distances between bony landmarks and adjacent nerves: anatomical factors that may influence retractor placement in total hip replacement surgery. J Orthop Surg 2016;11:31.

37. Macheras GA, Christofilopoulos P, Lepetsos P, et al. Nerve injuries in total HIP arthroplasty with a mini invasive anterior approach. HIP Int 2016;26:338–43.

38. Bodine SC. Peripheral nerve physiology, anatomy and pathology. Orthop Basic Sci 1994;378.

39. Sunderland S. Blood supply of the sciatic nerve and its popliteal divisions in man. Arch Neurol Psychiatry 1945;54:283–9.

40. Butt AJ, McCarthy T, Kelly IP, et al. Sciatic nerve palsy secondary to postoperative haematoma in primary total hip replacement. J Bone Joint Surg Br 2005;87:1465–7.

41. Goulding K, Beaulé PE, Kim PR, et al. Incidence of lateral femoral cutaneous nerve neuropraxia after anterior approach hip arthroplasty. Clin Orthop 2010;468:2397–404.

42. Hoshino C, Koga D, Koyano G, et al. Femoral nerve palsy following primary total hip arthroplasty with the direct anterior approach. PLOS ONE 2019;14:e0217068.

43. Moore AE, Stringer MD. Iatrogenic femoral nerve injury: a systematic review. Surg Radiol Anat 2011;33:649–58.

44. Ishimatsu T, Kinoshita K, Nishio J, et al. Motor-evoked potential analysis of femoral nerve status during the direct anterior approach for total hip arthroplasty. J Bone Jt Surg 2018;100:572–7.

45. Patton RS, Runner RP, Lyons RJ, et al. Clinical outcomes of patients with lateral femoral cutaneous nerve injury after direct anterior total hip arthroplasty. J Arthroplasty 2018;33:2919–26.e1.

46. McConaghie FA, Payne AP, Kinninmonth AWG. The role of retraction in direct nerve injury in total hip replacement: an anatomical study. Bone Jt Res 2014;3:212–6.

47. Yoshino K, Nakamura J, Hagiwara S, et al. Anatomical implications regarding femoral nerve palsy during a direct anterior approach to total hip arthroplasty: a cadaveric study. J Bone Jt Surg 2020;102:137–42.

48. Sullivan CW, Banerjee S, Desai K, et al. Safe zones for anterior acetabular retractor placement in direct anterior total hip arthroplasty: a cadaveric study. J Am Acad Orthop Surg 2019;27:e969–76.

49. Slater N, Singh R, Senasinghe N, et al. Pressure monitoring of the femoral nerve during total hip replacement: an explanation for iatropathic palsy. J R Coll Surg Edinb 2000;45:231–3.

50. Eggli S, Hankemayer S, Müller ME. Nerve palsy after leg lengthening in total replacement arthroplasty for developmental dysplasia of the hip. J Bone Joint Surg Br 1999;81:843–5.

51. Grob K, Manestar M, Ackland T, et al. Potential risk to the superior gluteal nerve during the anterior approach to the hip joint: an anatomical study. J Bone Jt Surg-am 2015;97:1426–31.

52. Jacobs LG, Buxton RA. The course of the superior gluteal nerve in the lateral approach to the hip. J Bone Joint Surg Am 1989;71:1239–43.

53. Eksioglu F, Uslu M, Gudemez E, et al. Reliability of the safe area for the superior gluteal nerve. Clin Orthop 2003;412:111–6.

54. Takada R, Jinno T, Miyatake K, et al. Direct anterior versus anterolateral approach in one-stage supine total hip arthroplasty. Focused on nerve injury: a prospective, randomized, controlled trial. J Orthop Sci 2018;23:783–7.

55. Putzer D, Haselbacher M, Hörmann R, et al. The distance of the gluteal nerve in relation to anatomical landmarks: an anatomic study. Arch Orthop Trauma Surg 2018;138:419–25.

56. Unis DB, Hawkins EJ, Alapatt MF, et al. Postoperative changes in the tensor fascia lata muscle after using the modified anterolateral approach for total hip arthroplasty. J Arthroplasty 2013;28:663–5.

57. Ince A, Kemper M, Waschke J, et al. Minimally invasive anterolateral approach to the hip: risk to the superior gluteal nerve. Acta Orthop 2007;78:86–9.

58. Abitbol JJ, Gendron D, Laurin CA, et al. Gluteal nerve damage following total hip arthroplasty. A prospective analysis. J Arthroplasty 1990;5:319–22.

59. Matta JM, Shahrdar C, Ferguson T. Single-incision anterior approach for total hip arthroplasty on an orthopaedic table. Clin Orthop Relat Res 2005; 441:115–24.

60. Meneghini RM, Pagnano MW, Trousdale RT, et al. Muscle damage during MIS total hip arthroplasty: Smith-Peterson versus posterior approach. Clin Orthop Relat Res 2006;453:293–8.

61. Kawasaki M, Hasegawa Y, Okura T, et al. Muscle damage after total hip arthroplasty through the direct anterior approach for developmental dysplasia of the hip. J Arthroplasty 2017;32:2466–73.

62. Rudin D, Manestar M, Ullrich O, et al. The anatomical course of the lateral femoral cutaneous nerve with special attention to the anterior approach to the hip joint. J Bone Jt Surg 2016;98:561–7.

63. Bartlett JD, Lawrence JE, Khanduja V. What is the risk posed to the lateral femoral cutaneous nerve during the use of the anterior portal of supine hip arthroscopy and the minimally invasive anterior approach for total hip arthroplasty? Arthrosc J Arthrosc Relat Surg 2018;34:1833–40.

64. Homma Y, Baba T, Sano K, et al. Lateral femoral cutaneous nerve injury with the direct anterior approach for total hip arthroplasty. Int Orthop 2016;40:1587–93.

65. Bhargava T, Goytia RN, Jones LC, et al. Lateral femoral cutaneous nerve impairment after direct anterior approach for total hip arthroplasty. Orthopedics 2010;33:472.

66. Ozaki Y, Homma Y, Baba T, et al. Spontaneous healing of lateral femoral cutaneous nerve injury and improved quality of life after total hip arthroplasty via a direct anterior approach: survey at average 12.8 and 26.2 months of follow-up. J Orthop Surg 2017;25. 230949901668475.

67. Kennon RE, Keggi JM, Wetmore RS, et al. Total hip arthroplasty through a minimally invasive anterior surgical approach. J Bone Jt Surg 2003;85:39–48.

68. Restrepo C, Parvizi J, Pour AE, et al. Prospective randomized study of two surgical approaches for total hip arthroplasty. J Arthroplasty 2010;25:671–9.e1.

69. Berend KR, Lombardi AV, Seng BE, et al. Enhanced early outcomes with the anterior supine intermuscular approach in primary total hip arthroplasty. J Bone Joint Surg Am 2009;91(Suppl 6):107–20.

70. Chen M, Luo Z, Ji X, et al. Direct anterior approach for total hip arthroplasty in the lateral decubitus position: our experiences and early results. J Arthroplasty 2017;32:131–8.

71. Ozaki Y, Homma Y, Sano K, et al. Small femoral offset is a risk factor for lateral femoral cutaneous nerve injury during total hip arthroplasty using a direct anterior approach. Orthop Traumatol Surg Res 2016;102:1043–7.

72. Elsaidi GA, Ruch DS, Schaefer WD, et al. Complications associated with traction on the hip during arthroscopy. J Bone Joint Surg Br 2004;86-B:793–6.

73. Pailhé R, Chiron P, Reina N, et al. Pudendal nerve neuralgia after hip arthroscopy: retrospective study and literature review. Orthop Traumatol Surg Res 2013;99:785–90.

74. Flierl MA, Stahel PF, Hak DJ, et al. Traction table-related complications in orthopaedic surgery. J Am Acad Orthop Surg 2010;18:668–75.

75. Siliski JM, Scott RD. Obturator-nerve palsy resulting from intrapelvic extrusion of cement during total hip replacement. Report of four cases. J Bone Jt Surg 1985;67:1225–8.

76. Unwin A, Scott J. Nerve palsy after hip replacement: medico-legal implications. Int Orthop 1999; 23:133–7.

77. Nercessian OA, Macaulay W, Stinchfield FE. Peripheral neuropathies following total hip arthroplasty. J Arthroplasty 1994;9:645–51.

78. Siguier T, Siguier M, Brumpt B. Mini-incision anterior approach does not increase dislocation rate: a study of 1037 total hip replacements. Clin Orthop 2004;164–73.

79. Hallert O, Li Y, Brismar H, et al. The direct anterior approach: initial experience of a minimally invasive technique for total hip arthroplasty. J Orthop Surg 2012;7:17.

80. Clawson DK, Seddon HJ. The late consequences of sciatic nerve injury. J Bone Joint Surg Br 1960;42: 213–25.

81. Pekkarinen J, Alho A, Puusa A, et al. Recovery of sciatic nerve injuries in association with total hip arthroplasty in 27 patients. J Arthroplasty 1999;14: 305–11.

82. Zappe B, Glauser PM, Majewski M, et al. Long-term prognosis of nerve palsy after total hip arthroplasty: results of two-year-follow-ups and long-term results after a mean time of 8 years. Arch Orthop Trauma Surg 2014;134:1477–82.

83. Lee G-C, Marconi D. Complications following direct anterior hip procedures: costs to both patients and surgeons. J Arthroplasty 2015;30: 98–101.

84. D'Arrigo C, Speranza A, Monaco E, et al. Learning curve in tissue sparing total hip replacement: comparison between different approaches. J Orthop Trauma 2009;10:47–54.

85. Hartog YM den, Vehmeijer SBW. High complication rate in the early experience of minimally invasive total hip arthroplasty by the direct anterior approach. Acta Orthop 2013;84:116–7.

Elevated Pre-operative D-Dimer Levels Do Not Impact the Effect of Tranexamic Acid on Revision Total Knee Arthroplasty

John M. Tarazi, MD[a,b], Theofanis P. Zois, PA[c],
Andrew Bohm, PhD[c], Michael A. Mont, MD[c,d,*],
Giles R. Scuderi, MD[b,c]

KEYWORDS

- D-dimer • Revision total knee arthroplasty • rTKA • Tranexamic acid • TXA

KEY POINTS

- The purpose of this study was to determine if elevated pre-operative D-dimer levels in patients undergoing rTKA pose an increased risk of: (1) post-operative venous thromboemboli (VTEs); (2) intra-operative blood loss; and (3) need for transfusion of blood products.
- Within the 90-day post-operative period, there were no VTE events identified in either cohort of patients.
- The mean drop in hemoglobin was similar for patients who had elevated D-dimer levels (2.05 g/dL) and those who had normal D-dimer levels (2.14 g/dL; $p = 0.28$). Likewise, the mean drop in hematocrit was similar for patients who had elevated D-dimer levels (5.44%) and those who had normal D-dimer levels (6.25%; $p = 0.13$). There were 2 patients (2.25%) who received transfusions, 1 patient in the normal D-dimer group and 1 patient in the elevated D-dimer group.

INTRODUCTION

D-dimer is a fibrin degradation by-product of blood clot breakdown that is not typically present in human plasma unless the coagulation system has been activated. Thus, during the formation of a thrombus, D-dimer assays become clinically useful when suspecting venous thromboemboli (VTEs) disorders that include pulmonary emboli (PEs) and deep vein thromboses (DVTs). There is recent evidence that serum D-dimer tests are promising for the diagnosis of peri-prosthetic joint infections (PJIs), but their true utility for this application is still controversial.[1–3] Nevertheless, patients who are candidates for revision total knee arthroplasty (rTKA) usually undergo plasma D-dimer testing to help determine whether the cause of primary arthroplasty failure was septic in nature.

It has been well documented that rTKA poses an increased risk of transfusion compared with primary TKA, with blood loss and subsequent transfusions following rTKA ranging between 30% and 62%.[4] Owing to the morbidity associated with perioperative anemia, surgeons strive to reduce perioperative blood loss. In doing so, antifibrinolytic agents such as tranexamic

[a] Department of Orthopaedics, Northwell Health—Huntington Hospital, 270 Park Avenue, Huntington, NY, 11743, USA; [b] Donald and Barbara Zucker School of Medicine at Hofstra/Northwell, 500 Hofstra Boulevard, Hempstead, NY, 11549, USA; [c] Department of Orthopaedics, Northwell Health—Lenox Hill Hospital, 130 East 77th Street, 11th Floor, Black Hall, New York, NY, 10075, USA; [d] Rubin Institute of Advanced Orthopedics, Center for Joint Preservation and Replacement, Sinai Hospital of Baltimore, 2401 West Belvedere Avenue, Baltimore, MD, 21215, USA
* Corresponding author.
E-mail address: Rhondamont@aol.com

Orthop Clin N Am 53 (2022) 139–143
https://doi.org/10.1016/j.ocl.2021.12.001
0030-5898/22/© 2021 Elsevier Inc. All rights reserved.

acid (TXA) have been used to reduce surgical blood loss and transfusion requirements following rTKA.[5–7] Furthermore, the safety of TXA has been well reported, and it acts by decreasing blood loss by inhibiting the ability of plasmin to break down fibrin, thereby decreasing blood clot dissolution, one of which includes D-dimer.

It became apparent to us that the effects of TXA on patients who have elevated D-dimer levels before rTKA were not clear. Specifically, there is a paucity of literature evaluating the rates of VTEs, blood loss, and transfusion requirements for these patients. Therefore, the purpose of this study was to determine if elevated pre-operative D-dimer levels in patients undergoing rTKA pose an increased risk of: (1) post-operative VTEs; (2) intra-operative blood loss; and (3) need for transfusion of blood products.

METHODS

Following institutional review board approval, a search was performed to identify all rTKAs performed by a single surgeon between January 1, 2017, and December 31, 2019. Inclusion criteria were revision of both femoral and tibial components for aseptic TKA failure and complete pre-operative serology testing including C-reactive protein (CRP), erythrocyte sedimentation rate (ESR), and D-dimer. A total of 89 cases met the inclusion criteria including 37 males (41.6%) and 52 females (58.4%). The mean age for males and females was 65 ± 10 years and 67 ± 10.5 years, respectively. The pre-operative serology data for each patient were recorded including D-dimer, ESR, and CRP.

All patients underwent complete revision of the femoral and tibial components with a cemented revision system under tourniquet control. All patients received peri-operative TXA following a standard protocol, 82 patients received 1 g intravenously (IV) before tourniquet inflation and 1 g before deflation, whereas 7 patients received intra-articular application of 2 g in 50 mL normal saline. The mode of prescribing TXA was based on institutional guidelines and agreed upon by the surgical team and anesthesia. All patients received 40 mg enoxaparin (Sanofi Aventis, USA) daily for 2 weeks following surgery followed by aspirin 325 mg twice per day for 4 weeks. The incidence of post-operative VTEs within the 90-day post-operative period was recorded, along with the change in pre-operative and post-operative hemoglobin and need for transfusion.

Statistical Analyses

All biomarkers in this study were evaluated as both continuous markers if possible and as dichotomous markers of "in acceptable range" and "out of acceptable range." This was necessary because some markers, such as hemoglobin, have acceptable ranges, which differ between genders. The reference concentration of D-dimer is less than 250 ng/mL, or less than 0.4 μg/mL (PAGANA National laboratory reference).[8] Owing to the way in which some values are stored in the electronic health record, some markers could only be evaluated dichotomously. t-tests were performed to evaluate for differences in continuous measures between patients with and without an elevated D-dimer level. Paired t-tests were conducted for evaluation of the change in hemoglobin, because this is the one biomarker included in the study that had both presurgical and postsurgical values. Chi-square tests were implemented, for "in range" and "out of range" dichotomous biomarkers, stratifying the population by D-dimer elevation status to evaluate for any significant differences. Testing was done following the same methods, but after stratifying the population by gender, there were not any systematic differences in study patients. All analyses were conducted using SPSS v. 25 (IBM, USA). The threshold for statistical significance was set to a p-value less than 0.05.

RESULTS

The pre-operative serology data were evaluated for all 89 patients. The data revealed that there were 54 patients (61%) who had an elevated D-dimer level and 35 patients (39%) who had a normal D-dimer level (Table 1). When stratified for sex, there were 21 males (57.8%) and 33 females (63.5%) who had an elevated D-dimer level ($p = 0.523$).

The mean drop in hemoglobin was similar for patients who had elevated D-dimer levels (2.05 g/dL) compared with those who had normal D-dimer levels (2.14 g/dL; $p = 0.28$). Likewise, the mean drop in hematocrit was similar for patients who had elevated D-dimer levels (5.44%) compared with those who had normal D-dimer levels (6.25%; $p = 0.13$). The mean pre-operative hemoglobin level was 13.3 ± 1.5 g/dL (range, 9.5–18.2 g/dL), and the mean post-operative hemoglobin level was 11.2 ± 1.4 g/dL (range, 7.7–13.8 g/dL). The mean pre-operative and post-operative hematocrit was $40.2\% \pm 4.3\%$ (range, 29.9%–55.2%) and $34.5\% \pm 3.9\%$ (range,

Table 1
Observed differences between groups

	Elevated D-Dimer	Normal D-Dimer	p-Value
N	54	35	
Male	21	16	0.52
Female	33	19	
Age	68.49	64.61	0.1
BMI	31.94	32.6	0.61
Mean hemoglobin drop (g/dL)	2.05	2.14	0.28
Mean hematocrit drop (%)	5.44	6.25	0.13
Transfusions	1	1	-
Venous thromboemboli	0	0	-

Abbreviation: BMI, body mass index.

25.3%–43.7%), respectively. Within the 90-day post-operative period, there were no VTE events identified in either cohort of patients.

There were 2 patients (2.25%) who received transfusions, 1 patient in the normal D-dimer group and 1 patient in the elevated D-dimer group (Table 2). Both patients received IV TXA. Although the number of patients receiving transfusions was small, it was noted that 1 patient had a preoperative hemoglobin level lower than that of the other 87 patients, whereas the second patient had a greater change in post-operative hemoglobin level (see Table 2). Statistical analysis was not performed because only 2 patients were transfused.

DISCUSSION

D-dimer assays are useful when there is clinical suspicion of VTEs. A negative D-dimer test essentially rules out a thrombosis, whereas a positive result can indicate thrombosis, but does not rule out other potential causes. Owing to its poor specificity, further testing is typically needed when elevated D-dimer results are encountered. There is recent evidence that serum D-dimer tests are promising for the diagnosis of PJIs,[10,11,15] but their true utility for this application is still controversial. Patients who are candidates for rTKA at our institution usually undergo plasma D-dimer testing to help determine if there is a PJI. As rTKAs have been associated with substantial blood loss and

subsequent post-operative transfusions, TXA has been proved to be an effective tool in the prevention of blood loss and transfusion following primary and revision procedures. The results of our study demonstrated that within 90 days of rTKA, no VTE events occurred in patients who had normal or elevated D-dimer levels. In addition, there were no differences in blood loss between groups as evidenced by post-operative changes in hemoglobin or hematocrit.

This study is not without limitations. Owing to our relatively small sample size, our results may be subject to type II error. That is, although we did not identify differences in our measured outcomes between groups, a larger sample size may be required to demonstrate no differences between patients who have normal and elevated D-dimer levels. However, this is the first study to evaluate this research question, and it may pave the way for future large-scale studies investigating this topic. The other limitation of the study is that it reports the post-operative VTE events only within a 90-day episode of care. However, we feel that this is a critical time interval for the prevention of VTE events. Owing to the relatively low incidence of VTEs following joint arthroplasty, it is critical to apply this research question to a larger patient population to accept the null hypotheses.

There are concerns with the use of TXA in patients who have an increased risk of blood clotting or history of VTEs, PEs, or DVTs, thus these comorbidities have been identified as contraindications to its use. Antifibrinolytic agents such as TXA decrease blood loss by inhibiting the ability of plasmin to break down fibrin, thereby acting to decrease clot dissolution.[9] D-dimer is a product of blood clot dissolution, and for this reason, it has been used as an initial screening test for patients who have signs and symptoms of VTE.

In evaluating the results of D-dimer testing, it is essential to assess the clinical probability of diagnosing a VTE. In patients who have a low, intermediate, or high clinical probability, the clinical prevalence of DVT with an elevated D-dimer is less than 5%, 15%, and 70%, respectively, whereas the prevalence of PE was 8%, 28%, and 74%, respectively.[10,11] This patient profiling is important because many factors impact the sensitivity and specificity of D-dimer testing, including the extent of the thrombosis and fibrinolytic activity, duration of symptoms, anticoagulant therapy, comorbidity due to surgical or medical illnesses, inflammatory diseases, cancer, elderly age, pregnancy and puerperium,

Table 2
Patient transfusion (statistical analysis not performed because only 2 patients transfused)

	Age (y)	Sex	Pre-operative Hgb (g/dL)	Post-operative Hgb (g/dL)	Change in Hgb (g/dL)
Patient 1	63	Female	12.8	7.8	5.0
Patient 2	54	Female	11.2	9.0	2.2
Total cohort	Age (mean)	Female (%)	Mean pre-operative Hgb (g/dL)	Mean post-operative Hgb (g/dL)	Mean change in Hgb (g/dL)
Transfused (n = 2)	58.5	100	12.0	8.4	3.6
Nontransfused (n = 87)	66.1	57.47	13.3	11.3	2.1

Abbreviation: Hgb, hemoglobin.

increasing age (>65 years), African American heritage, cigarette smoking, recent trauma, and previous VTE.[12,13]

Numerous studies have also shown that systemic and local infections result in fibrinolytic activities, and D-dimer has gained attention for its role in predicting the outcome of sepsis and bacteremia.[3,14,15,16] Serum D-dimer has also been shown to be a marker for the diagnosis of PJIs and has been recommended by the Musculoskeletal Infection Society (MSIS) to be a test for patients undergoing a workup for PJIs.[3]

Despite the elevated D-dimer levels in 54 patients (63%) who underwent rTKA in this study, there was not an increased incidence of VTE. The presence of an elevated preoperative D-dimer level in the evaluation of a failed TKA, pending revision, should not necessarily be considered a contraindication to the use of TXA during surgery.

In this study the authors concluded that: (1) an elevated preoperative D-dimer level is not a contraindication to the use of TXA; (2) an elevated preoperative D-dimer level did not pose an increased risk of post-operative VTEs; and (3) TXA is effective in reducing blood loss following rTKA.

SUMMARY

The authors of this study are the first to evaluate whether elevated preoperative D-dimer level impacts the effect of TXA on rTKA. Despite the relatively small sample size, this study may pave the way for future large-scale studies investigating this topic. Furthermore, larger sample sizes may be required to demonstrate no differences between patients who have normal and elevated D-dimer levels. The authors of this

study concluded that: (1) an elevated preoperative D-dimer level is not a contraindication to the use of TXA; (2) an elevated preoperative D-dimer did not pose an increased risk of post-operative VTEs; and (3) TXA is effective in reducing blood loss following rTKA.

CLINICS CARE POINTS

- Elevated pre-operative D-dimer did not pose an increased risk of VTE, blood loss, or transfusion of blood products.
- These results are important because they demonstrate that elevated pre-operative D-dimer is not a contraindication to the use of TXA for revision total knee arthroplasty.

DISCLOSURE

M.A. Mont is a board or committee member for The Knee Society and The Hip Society, receives research support from National Institutes of Health, and is on the editorial board for the Journal of Arthroplasty, Journal of Knee Surgery, Surgical Technology International, and Orthopaedics. He also receives company support from 3M, Centrexion, Ceras Health, Flexion Therapeutics, Johnson & Johnson, Kolon TissueGene, NXSCI, US Medical Innovations, Pacira, Pfizer-Lily, Skye Biologics, SOLVD Health, Smith and Nephew, Stryker, CERAS Health, MirrorAR, Peerwell, US Medical Innovations, Johnson & Johnson, RegenLab, TissueGene, Stryker, MedicusWorks LLC, Up-to Date, Wolters Kluwer Health–Lippincott Williams & Wilkins, Journal of Arthroplasty, Journal of Knee Surgery, Orthopedics, Surgical Techniques International; AAHKS, Knee

Society, and Hip Society. Dr Giles R. Scuderi receives royalties and/or is a consultant for Zimmer Biomet, 3M KCI, Elsevier, Springer, Thieme, and World Scientific. He has stock options in Force Therapeutics and ROM Tech. G.R. Scuderi is also on the editorial board for the Journal of Knee Surgery and is a board member for Operation Walk USA. All other authors have no conflicts of interest to disclose.

REFERENCES

1. Pannu TS, Villa JM, Riesgo AM, et al. Serum D-Dimer in the diagnosis of periprosthetic knee infection: where are we today? J Knee Surg 2020;33(2):106–10.

2. Parvizi J, Tan TL, Goswami K, et al. The 2018 definition of periprosthetic hip and knee infection: an evidence-based and validated criteria. J Arthroplasty 2018;33(5):1309–14.e2.

3. Shahi A, Kheir MM, Tarabichi M, et al. Serum D-Dimer test is promising for the diagnosis of periprosthetic joint infection and timing of reimplantation. J Bone Joint Surg Am 2017;99(17):1419–27.

4. Sehat KR, Evans RL, Newman JH. Hidden blood loss following hip and knee arthroplasty. Correct management of blood loss should take hidden loss into account. J Bone Joint Surg Br 2004;86(4):561–5.

5. Fillingham YA, Darrith B, Calkins TE, et al. 2019 Mark Coventry Award: a multicentre randomized clinical trial of tranexamic acid in revision total knee arthroplasty: does the dosing regimen matter? Bone Joint J 2019;101-b(7_Supple_C):10–6.

6. Fillingham YA, Ramkumar DB, Jevsevar DS, et al. The efficacy of tranexamic acid in total knee arthroplasty: a network meta-analysis. J Arthroplasty 2018;33(10):3090–8.e1.

7. Fillingham YA, Ramkumar DB, Jevsevar DS, et al. The safety of tranexamic acid in total joint arthroplasty: a direct meta-analysis. J Arthroplasty 2018;33(10):3070–82.e1.

8. Hultin S. Mosby's manual of diagnostic and laboratory tests (4th edn). Ann Clin Biochem Int J Lab Med 2012. https://doi.org/10.1258/acb.2012.201207.

9. Dunn CJ, Goa KL. Tranexamic acid: a review of its use in surgery and other indications. Drugs 1999;57(6):1005–32.

10. Le Gal G, Righini M, Roy PM, et al. Prediction of pulmonary embolism in the emergency department: the revised Geneva score. Ann Intern Med 2006;144(3):165–71.

11. Wells PS, Anderson DR, Bormanis J, et al. Value of assessment of pretest probability of deep-vein thrombosis in clinical management. Lancet 1997;350(9094):1795–8.

12. Prisco D, Grifoni E. The role of D-dimer testing in patients with suspected venous thromboembolism. Semin Thromb Hemost 2009;35(1):50–9.

13. Pulivarthi S, Gurram MK. Effectiveness of d-dimer as a screening test for venous thromboembolism: an update. N Am J Med Sci 2014;6(10):491–9.

14. Gando S. Role of fibrinolysis in sepsis. Semin Thromb Hemost 2013;39(4):392–9.

15. Gris JC, Bouvier S, Cochery-Nouvellon E, et al. Fibrin-related markers in patients with septic shock: individual comparison of D-dimers and fibrin monomers impacts on prognosis. Thromb Haemost 2011;106(6):1228–30.

16. Michelin E, Snijders D, Conte S, et al. Procoagulant activity in children with community acquired pneumonia, pleural effusion and empyema. Pediatr Pulmonol 2008;43(5):472–5.

Trauma

Radial Nerve Injury in Humeral Shaft Fracture

Michael Daly, MD, Chris Langhammer, MD, PHD*

KEYWORDS

- Radial nerve injury • Humeral shaft fracture • Nerve repair

KEY POINTS

- Orthopedic surgeons should understand the principles of radial nerve injuries in the context of humeral shaft fractures in order to facilitate optimal treatment of this injury constellation.
- Expectant management of nerve injury in conjunction with nonoperative treatment of fracture includes appropriately timed clinical follow-up with detailed clinical examinations and serial electromyograms.
- Surgical exploration (with possible reconstruction) is recommended at 3 to 4 months from injury if there is no evidence of improvement.
- Treatment of radial nerve injuries identified at the time of operatively treated fractures includes direct repair under no tension when possible, reconstruction with graft if repair is not possible, and tagging the nerve ends under physiologic tension with referral for specialist care when acute reconstruction is not appropriate.
- Irreparable proximal radial nerve injuries benefit from distal nerve or tendon transfers.

INTRODUCTION

Fractures of the humeral shaft are common, accounting for 1% to 3% of all fractures.[1] Concurrent radial nerve injury has been reported in approximately 10% of these fractures.[2] Certain fracture patterns may carry an even higher incidence of radial nerve injury. The classic example of this is a spiral fracture at the distal third of the humeral diaphysis, otherwise known as the Holstein-Lewis fracture.[3]

At the time of initial presentation, the extent to which the nerve is damaged is often unknown, but the mechanism itself can provide clues as to the nature of the nerve injury. However, any injury pattern is capable of creating the whole spectrum of nerve injuries from contusion to complete transection. For example, open injuries with a sharp penetrating mechanism are classically thought to have a higher likelihood of nerve transection secondary to the laceration of soft tissues within the field of injury. Ballistic injuries are classically thought to have a higher likelihood of nerve contusion secondary to the shock-wave and soft tissue contusion caused by the high-velocity projectile. Closed humeral shaft fractures with simple fracture patterns can result in stretching of the nerve by displacement of the soft tissues at the time of injury, contusion of the nerve from entrapment between mobile fracture ends, or complete laceration of the nerve over the sharp edges of the fractured bone.[4,5]

Treatment algorithms are designed around reducing the overall time to appropriate treatment in the context of this uncertainty. An understanding of the treatment for these injuries is enriched by an understanding of the anatomy, classification, and prognosis for peripheral nerve injuries generally.

Peripheral Nerve Injury

The microstructural anatomy of the peripheral nervous system is most usefully conceptualized as a series of concentric layers from the inside

Department of Orthopaedic Traumatology, University of Maryland, 22 South Greene Street, Baltimore, MD 21201, USA
* Corresponding author.
E-mail address: clanghammer@som.umaryland.edu

Orthop Clin N Am 53 (2022) 145–154
https://doi.org/10.1016/j.ocl.2022.01.001

to the outside (Fig. 1A).[6] The basic unit of the peripheral nervous system is the single axon, which conducts action potentials, as a means of neurotransmission. An interrupted myelin sheath surrounds the axon, accelerating conduction velocity. The endoneurial lining surrounds these 2 elements and is the peripheral analogue to the "blood-brain barrier" in the central nervous system. Functional axonal units with similar function are clustered into fascicles by the perineurium, from which peripheral nerves derive their tensile strength. Fascicles for specific anatomic regions are clustered into named peripheral nerves by the epineurium, which houses the vasonervosum (the blood supply for the peripheral nervous system).

There are 2 classification systems for peripheral nervous system injury, which are both based on this underlying anatomic arrangement (Fig. 1B). The Sunderland classification system is based on the microstructural level of injury.[7] The 5 levels of peripheral nervous system microstructure include the following: I, mylin sheath; II, axon; III, endoneurium; IV, perineurium; V, epineurium. Ascending levels of injury in the Sunderland classification system represent disruption of the corresponding microstructural element listed above, along with all of the preceding microstructural elements.

The Sedon classification system consists of 3 levels (neurapraxia, axonotmesis, and neurotmesis) and is based on function and macroscopic anatomy (see Fig. 1B).[8] Neuropraxia represents a transient disruption in nerve conduction most commonly thought to be secondary to temporary disruption of the myelin sheath (Sunderland grade I). Axonotmesis is any injury disrupting the axon, without disrupting the macroscopic continuity of the peripheral nerve as seen from the outside (Sunderland grade II, III, and IV). Neurotmesis is an injury causing frank discontinuity of the peripheral nerve (Sunderland grade V).[9]

Recovery of appropriate action potential conduction across a region of injury depends on the severity of the injury. Neuropraxia has an excellent prognosis, as no axonal regeneration is required. The prognosis of axonotmetic injury depends largely on the level of microstructural disruption. Axonotmetic injuries preserving the microstructure allow regenerating axons to reliably find their original target and have good prognoses without surgical intervention. Axonotmetic injuries with disruption of microstructure do not allow for successful nerve regrowth and have poor nonsurgical outcomes. The exercise of trying to determine the difference in severity of axonotmetic injuries is largely intellectual, as this is practically indeterminable outside of research laboratories. Last, neurotmetic injuries will not recover without surgical intervention.

A good clinical outcome after nerve injury depends on the likelihood that nerve conduction will be restored from its origin to its intended target before that intended target undergoes atrophy, loss of function, and cellular death. This means that prognosis for recovery of native nerve function depends on the nature of injury according to the injury classification system above, as well as other features of the host and injury (Fig. 1C).[10,11] Younger patients with greater regenerative potential, both centrally and peripherally, carry a better prognosis. Injuries occurring distally in an extremity carry a better prognosis because axonal growth cones have a shorter distance to traverse before finding their target and successful reinnervation of target end plates. Injuries requiring surgical intervention that are repaired earlier carry a better prognosis because early intervention reduces the time to reinnervation. Injuries that can be repaired directly (end to end) carry a better prognosis because regenerating nerves only have 1 coaptation to navigate, rather than having 2 coaptation sites as is the case with any grafting technique.

PATIENT EVALUATION AND CLINICAL DECISION MAKING

Each of the patient and injury factors affecting prognosis do so by affecting the time to

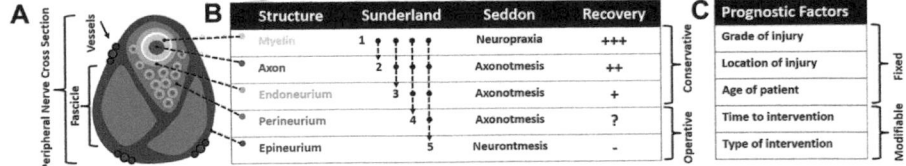

Fig. 1. Peripheral nerve injury primer. (A) Overview of peripheral nerve anatomy as mapped onto (B) Sunderland and Sedon injury classification systems and association with prognosis. (C) Additional factors driving outcomes in peripheral nerve injury.

reinnervation or extent of reinnervation. A good clinical outcome depends on the likelihood that nerve conduction will be restored from its origin to its intended target before the intended target dies. In the case of the neuromuscular junction, end organ death is thought to occur approximately 12 months from denervation (Fig. 2).[11] This means that selecting the most appropriate treatment pathway requires a timely decision to proceed with surgery when it becomes necessary. It is the surgeon's obligation to identify patients for whom expectant management is unlikely to succeed and indicate them for early corrective intervention.

Expectant Management

Expectant management consists of serial examinations (detailed physical examination and electromyogram [EMG]), timed in such a way to catch the leading edge of clinical recovery (see Fig. 2C). Evidence of early returning function rules out neurotmetic injuries that would benefit from early exploration with reconstruction. Radial nerve injuries in the context of humeral shaft fractures are expected to recover without intervention in more than 70% of cases, and approximately 90% of cases, including those that underwent procedural intervention.[12] In the context of closed fractures, recovery with expectant management is even more likely,[4,5,13] with recovery rates consistently greater than 90%.

Physical examination

The pattern of muscle innervation of the radial nerve is reproducible (Fig. 3).[14] The most common site of laceration is at the lateral margin of the humerus, where the radial nerve passes from the posterior compartment to the anterior compartment (see Fig. 3, point E). Nerve mobility is limited here secondary to tethering by the intermuscular septum, making it especially prone to neurotmetic injury. The most proximal motor endplates occur in the brachioradialis (BR) and extensor carpi radialis longus (ECRL; 10 cm and 12 cm from the lateral intermuscular septum, respectively). With an average regeneration rate of 1 mm/d, this implies that clinical evidence of recovery consisting of activation of the BR and ECRL should be observable by approximately 3.5 to 4.5 months from injury. After this point, reinnervation occurs in a reproducible pattern based on injury consisting of recovery of wrist extension, then extension over the ulnar-sided digits, and finally, extension of the thumb and index finger. Once reinnervation has started down this pathway, it generally restores good function in all muscle groups. However, very distal muscles, such as the extensor indicis proprius, with a reinnervation distance of 30 cm, are likely to take up to 10 months to recover. These calculated estimations of activity recovery are echoed in clinic observations of recovery in Sedon neuropraxic- and axonotmetic-type injuries, with early recovery noted by 12 months, and full recovery taking up to 1 year.[13] Additional early findings indicating that the nerve injury is not complete include preservation of sensory function. Motor function is the first to be lost and last to be regained after neuropraxic injury; incomplete injuries that preserve sensory function have an excellent prognosis. Similarly, advancing Tinel sign at the lateral aspect of the humerus during their initial visits carries an excellent prognosis, as it indicates regeneration down the distal portion of the nerve has already begun. Documentation of the exact location of the Tinel sign (single

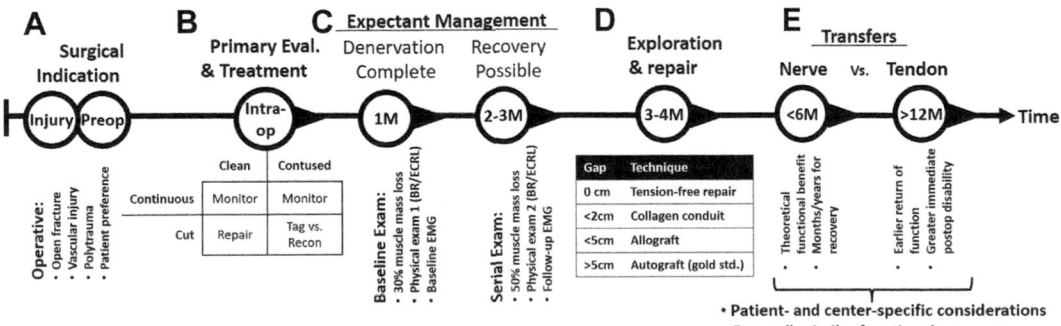

Fig. 2. Timeline of possible interventions with key points: decisions to proceed with intervention occur at multiple timepoints, including (A) primary surgical indications for fracture fixation, (B) intraoperative decision making regarding associated nerve injury, (C) expectant management, which may progress to (D) secondary exploration and reconstruction, and the possibility of (E) late nerve or tendon transfers. Eval., evaluation; Intra, intraoperative; Preop, preoperative; Postop, postoperative; Recon, reconstruction; Std., standard.

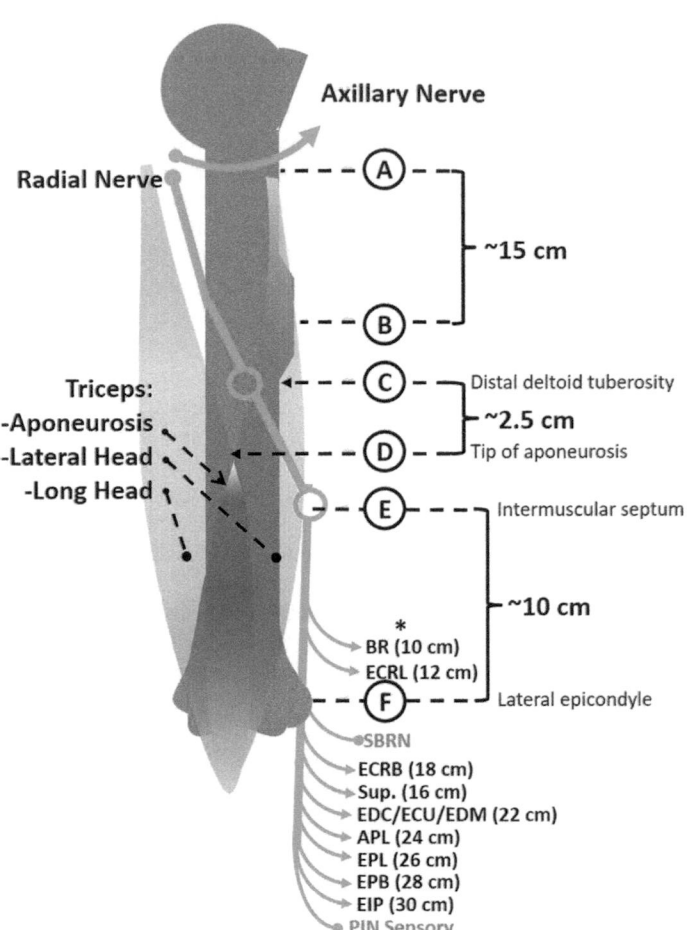

Axillary Nerve

Radial Nerve

A

~15 cm

B

C — Distal deltoid tuberosity

~2.5 cm

Triceps:
-Aponeurosis
-Lateral Head
-Long Head

D — Tip of aponeurosis

E — Intermuscular septum

~10 cm

*
BR (10 cm)
ECRL (12 cm)
F — Lateral epicondyle
●SBRN
ECRB (18 cm)
Sup. (16 cm)
EDC/ECU/EDM (22 cm)
APL (24 cm)
EPL (26 cm)
EPB (28 cm)
EIP (30 cm)
● PIN Sensory

Fig. 3. Radial nerve schematic with landmarks: radial nerve anatomy with relevant landmarks. APL, abductor pollicis longus; ECU, extensor carpi ulnaris; EDM, extensor digiti minimi; EIP, extensor indicis proprius; EPB, extensor pollicis brevis; EPL, extensor pollicis longus; PIN, posterior interosseous nerve; Sup., supinator. * indicates that the starting point of reinnervation after injury at the intermuscular septum.

spot with maximum effect) relative to the lateral epicondyle will help differentiate between patients with progressive recovery versus those with static neuroma formation.

Electromyogram

In cases whereby neurotmesis has occurred, no functional recovery will be observed. Clinically, this will appear simply as the absence of functional recovery over serial examinations. However, changes occur on the level of muscle cell function that may become evident while awaiting clinical improvement. Because the grade of the injury in unexplored cases cannot be known before initiating expectant management, serial EMGs are a useful way of providing additional quantitative measures of nerve function to supplement serial clinical examinations. A review of the EMG changes exceeds the scope of this review. However, these EMGs should be performed in the radial nerve innervated muscle groups listed previously specifically to assess

for progressive reinnervation or its absence. It is useful to have serial studies performed by the same provider and in the same location in order to allow for direct comparison of serial examinations. EMG changes, such as the development of abnormal spontaneous activity, are expected to evolve during the first 4 weeks after injury. EMG studies before this point are not recommended. A second EMG study at 3 to 4 months from injury will allow adequate time for most injuries to reach the proximal ECRL and BR in the case of axonotmetic injuries. In medicolegal cases, more frequent EMGs starting before this point may help identify the most likely timing of nerve injury, but this is not routinely recommended.[15,16]

Primary Exploration and Treatment of Nerve Injury

Indications for acute surgical exploration, with possible repair, are similar to indications for operative treatment of humeral shaft fractures;

these are (1) open fractures, (2) fractures complicated by vascular injury, (3) global patient injury constellations requiring fracture fixation with the theoretic benefit of earlier mobilization of the extremity, or (4) strong patient preference for operative treatment and an understanding of the associated risks and benefits (see **Fig. 2**A).

In the case of radial nerve injury, open reduction with internal fixation of the humeral shaft may be preferred over closed intramedullary nailing when the skeletal injury is amenable to both, for the simple reason that the nerve should be directly examined in these cases. There is a risk that the nerve palsy is secondary to incarceration in the fracture site, in which case the act of reaming and passing an intramedullary nail could cause secondary injury to the nerve.[17] In addition, minimally invasive surgical treatment is a missed opportunity to characterize the nerve injury, which assists with downstream clinical decision making. Surgical exploration of the fracture with visualization of the radial nerve should be at least considered when surgical fixation is indicated, regardless of skeletal fixation tactic.[13]

If a transected radial nerve is encountered during surgical fixation of a fracture, treatment of the radial nerve at that time depends on the continuity of the nerve (cut vs continuous), and the quality of the nerve (contused vs clean) (see **Fig. 2**B).

Continuous and clean

In cases whereby the nerve is in continuity and healthy-appearing, conservative management is expected to yield an excellent result, with recovery of full manual strength by 1 year from injury in 98% of cases.[13] In cases of nerve discontinuity or significant contusion, the prognosis is less clear, and there is little definitive evidence guiding clinical decision making.

Cut and clean

Cases whereby the nerve is cut and the ends are clean appearing may best be described as simple lacerations. The gold-standard treatment of any simple nerve laceration is direct, tension-free repair. Direct nerve repair falls generally into 2 categories: epineurial versus fascicular repair. Epineurial repairs consist of reapproximating of the epineurium using blood vessels and other surface landmarks to grossly restore alignment. The goal is to preserve fascicular alignment while limiting intraneural suture in an effort to reduce foreign body reaction and disordered scar formation at the coaptation site. Fascicular repair is the direct repair of individual fascicles, achieving direct fascicular realignment at the expense of increased manipulation of the nerve tissue and intraneural placement of sutures. In nerve repairs, as in nerve transfers, it is generally agreed that fascicular alignment is important.[18,19] However, the literature has not demonstrated the superiority of either of the above techniques.[20]

Regardless of the technique used, nerve repair should always be performed under no tension. The simplest way of achieving a tension-free repair is immobilization along the length of the proximal and distal nerve ends. Additional length can be achieved through anterior transposition of the nerve through the fracture site if fracture morphology and soft tissue injury patterns are amenable to this.

Continuous and contused

Nerves in gross continuity, but with a contused appearance, have the most variable prognosis. The epineurium is intact, but the internal extent of microstructural disruption is highly variable. In some cases, there is little disruption, and recovery progresses well. In other cases, the internal derangement prevents any effective axonal regrowth through the zone of injury and results in a neuroma-in-continuity. The long-term outcome is unknowable based on features available during visual inspection. Acute resection with grafting may be beneficial in a well-demarcated, short-segment crush injury. Otherwise, results with resection and grafting of a contused nerve in continuity may not yield better results than expectant management alone.

Cut and contused

Cases whereby the nerve is lacerated and the nerve ends appear contused are the most controversial. The first step generally requires the debridement of the injured-appearing nerve back to the level of healthy-appearing nerve fascicles. Many nerve surgeons advocate for performing this acutely. However, there has yet to be an objective way to identify and differentiate between contused portions of nerve that will recover versus a contused portion of nerve that will not recover. Some surgeons therefore advocate for tagging the nerve with the intention of performing a subacute reconstruction after the zone of nerve injury has been demarcated.

If definitive management of the nerve ends is not being performed at the initial surgical setting, classic teaching recommends tagging the free nerve ends proximally and distally with suture for easier identification later by the treating surgeon. It is the authors' viewpoint however that this technique is of limited utility. Simple suture tags do not prevent retraction of the nerve ends, and retraction of ~1.5 cm at each nerve end can be expected over the following weeks, resulting in a large nerve gap (Fig. 4C, blue bracket). In addition, free suture tags do not facilitate retrieval during secondary procedures, as they are difficult to identify within their surrounding scar tissue (see Fig. 4C, blue arrowheads). The authors' preferred tactic is suturing the nerve ends to one another under physiologic tension in order to prevent further retraction, preserve their alignment, and maintain the nerve's anatomic position to facilitate identification during subsequent reconstructive surgery. Some surgeons even recommend tagging the nerve ends with a collagen nerve tube. Staining the nerve tube with methylene blue to facilitate location of the nerve ends during a secondary procedure is another described approach. Regardless of the management choice, of critical importance are clear communication and documentation of the manner in which the nerve was addressed. A clear description of the

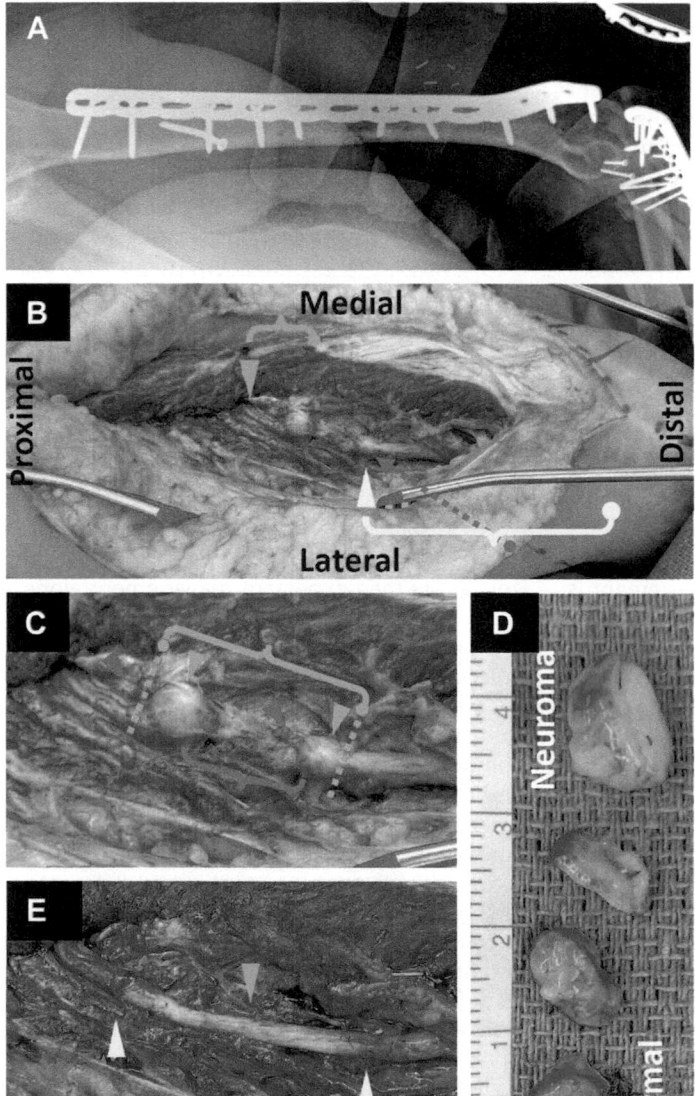

Fig. 4. Case example, delayed radial nerve reconstruction: A 38-year-old woman sustained an open humeral shaft fracture and transolecranon fracture dislocation in conjunction with a closed head injury complicated by ischemic stroke. She was medically stabilized, and a traumatic radial nerve transection was noted during index fixation of her humeral shaft fracture (A). The ends were tagged with 6-0 Prolene suture and left. The patient was referred for specialist care ~3 months after fixation for evaluation and treatment of her radial nerve injury. Surgical exposure consisted of a revision Gerwin approach consisting of elevation of the atretic lateral head of the triceps. The proximal portion of the radial nerve (B; green arrowhead) was found crossing the midpoint of the humerus 2 cm proximal to the tip of the triceps aponeurosis (B; green bracket). The distal portion of the nerve was found crossing the lateral aspect of the humerus (B; yellow arrowhead), 10 cm proximal to the lateral epicondyle (B; yellow bracket), where the proximal extension of the anterior forearm musculature had been marked on the skin with the elbow flexed 45° (B; blue dashed arrow). The nerve ends had formed neuroma (C; green arrowheads), which obscured the tagging suture (C; blue arrowheads). The unsecured nerve ends had retracted ~2 cm (C; blue bracket), almost doubling the total nerve gap after neuroma resection (C; green bracket). The proximal and distal neuromas were resected in sections until healthy-appearing fascicles were visualized (D). The resultant 4.5-cm gap was bridged using acellular allograft (E; green arrowhead) rather than autograft at the patient's request, and to coaptation sites were reinforced with a nerve wrap (E; yellow arrowheads).

location of the laceration and the fate of the discontinuous nerve ends, as well as a description of the approximate location of the nerve relative to any fixation can additionally be useful to receiving surgeons, especially if the nerve was left in an extra-anatomic position.

There is no evidence-based guidance on the timing of secondary nerve reconstruction, with recommendations ranging from 3 days to 3 weeks.[21] It is the authors' experience that early reoperations within 1 week of the index surgery simplify the process of isolating the nerve ends, whereas delayed reoperations performed more than 3 weeks from injury simplify identification of the zone of injury. These treatment decisions should be made by the surgeon who will ultimately perform the surgery, however, so referral to a specialist as soon as possible is critically important in optimizing patient care.

Secondary Nerve Exploration and Reconstruction

Secondary surgical exploration of radial nerve injuries, which have not improved with expectant management, is most commonly performed between 3 and 5 months from injury. Indication for surgery includes the absence of any clinical or EMG evidence of recovering function (see Fig. 2D).[12] This time period allows for the development of any early observable clinical recovery in nerves that will recover native function and allows for the earliest possible exploration of the zone of nerve injury in nerves that will not. If an injury requiring proximal reconstruction is found and repaired, this timing allows for 8 months of regeneration following repair before reaching the 12-month deadline at which loss of neuromuscular junctions becomes irreversible. Secondary reoperation in cases of known transection should be performed as soon as the soft tissues and patient are amenable to a second surgery.

Operating through healthy tissue planes is always ideal but is frequently not possible in the context of secondary exploration. A knowledge of the previous approach used for skeletal fixation (ie, if a Gerwin approach vs a triceps splitting approach was used) may help establish an expectation of which tissue planes may remain useful during reexposure of the radial nerve.

The authors recommend using a Gerwin approach, including elevation of the lateral head of the triceps off the intermuscular septum.[22] This approach is advantageous because the location for nerve injury is often at its transition point from the posterior to anterior compartment (see Fig. 3, point E). In cases whereby a triceps-splitting approach was used

for skeletal fixation, the lateral tissue plane may even be preserved, facilitating the dissection and exposure of the radial nerve. The lower lateral cutaneous sensory nerve can be followed through the lateral head of the triceps to the radial nerve. However, during revision exposures, this anatomic landmark may not be as readily identifiable. In cases where the Gerwin approach was used at the index procedure (Fig. 4A), it may be possible to find motor branches to the lateral head of the triceps during its reelevation, which can be followed to the proximal stump of the radial nerve. If the location of injury is more proximal or the lateral triceps cannot be safely reelevated, the radial nerve can be found proximally between the long and lateral head of the triceps in the triangular window (see Fig. 3, points A–B).

If clean tissue planes cannot be established and followed to the region of nerve injury, gross anatomic musculoskeletal landmarks can be used. The proximal segment of the radial nerve most frequently crosses the midpoint of the humeral shaft at the level of the distal end of the deltoid tuberosity radiographically (see Fig. 3, point C). This same point can be located immediately deep to a point 2 cm proximal to the proximal-most tip of the triceps aponeurosis (see Fig. 3, points C–D; see Fig. 4B, green bracket).

The distal segment of the radial nerve crosses the humerus laterally at a point 10 cm proximal to the lateral epicondyle (see Fig. 3, point E; see Fig 4B, yellow bracket). The same point can be identified by placing the elbow at 45° of flexion and marking a line indicating a proximal extension of the anterior aspect of the forearm musculature (see Fig. 4B, blue line and blue dots). This line approximates the anterior edge of the BR, and its intersection with the humerus indicates where the radial nerve passes between the BR and the brachialis muscle bellies at the lateral aspect of the humerus.

Once the nerve segments have been found proximally and distally, they can be followed reliably into the zone of injury, exposing the neuromata at their ends (see Fig. 4C, green arrowheads). The neuroma tissue prevents ordered nerve regrowth and therefore needs to be trimmed to the level of healthy-appearing fascicles in order to facilitate a functional repair. The "bread-loafing" technique is commonly described in this setting. Thin cross-sections are taken in the direction of diseased tissue toward healthy tissue and examined at each section for the appearance of the fascicles (see Fig. 4D). Sectioning is stopped when normal-appearing fascicles are reached. Healthy fascicular ends are an absolute requirement for nerve regeneration. However, reducing the amount of resected tissue to only the required amount to reach this level is important in limiting the net nerve gap. The final nerve gap (see Fig. 4C, green bracket) is the sum of the gap created by nerve end retraction (see Fig. 4C, blue bracket) and additional proximal and distal tissue loss from neuroma resection (see Fig. 4C, green arrowheads). The size of the defect can be mitigated through proximal and distal mobilization of the nerve (or even nerve transposition, as mentioned previously) in order to simplify subsequent reconstructive steps.

The technique used to bridge the resultant gap between cleaned nerve ends depends on the gap size. Optimal techniques to facilitate nerve regeneration across the gap, especially with regards to autograft versus the increasingly popular option of acellular allograft, remain controversial. However, classic teaching would dictate the following general guidelines: nerve gaps less than 3 cm can be bridged effectively using a collagen conduit; nerve gaps less than 5 cm can be bridged effectively using acellular allograft (see Fig. 4E, green arrowhead); and nerve gaps greater than 5 cm require autogenous graft.[23] Adjunct techniques consisting of a variety of nerve wraps or other neuroprotective implantables (see Fig. 4E, blue arrowheads) are becoming increasingly popular; however, data supporting any technique over any other technique remain limited.

Tendon and Nerve Transfers

In cases whereby the proximal defect is irreparable or the time window for direct repair has been missed, distal nerve transfers or tendon transfers offer an extra-anatomic set of reconstructive tools. The outcomes for these procedures are consistently good in the context of radial nerve injuries,[24] prompting some groups to promote nerve and tendon transfers over primary repair as the treatment of choice regardless of the time or nature of injury. In addition, combination surgeries using both nerve and tendon transfers to provide a mix of their respective benefits are becoming popular, blurring the lines between these 2 treatment avenues.[25]

All transfer surgeries require removing functionality from one source in order to replace functionality that has been lost someplace else. The details of each transfer sequence are designed to reduce the donor site morbidity and expedite the postoperative return of function to the recipient site by matching magnitude and direction of activity (synergistic transfers).

An overview of the unique pros and cons of a nerve transfer surgery versus tendon transfer surgery is discussed briefly in later discussion. There is continued debate regarding outcomes from these procedures, with some case series reporting superiority of the more recently developed nerve transfers,[26] and some reporting equivalence.[25] Interpretation of these results is complicated by the limited number of centers publishing on this topic, the tremendous selection bias in these retrospective studies, and the differences in technique and reporting used between studies.

Nerve transfers

Donor nerves are selected that are redundant (have multiple motor pedicles or multiple muscle groups with overlapping function), are size matched to the recipient nerves, are locally available to the recipient nerve, and exist in a host with excellent neuroregenerative capacity (young age). Nerve transfers for high radial nerve injury require the sacrifice of nerve branches from the median nerve to supplement radial nerve branches. The most commonly used is transfer of a flexor digitorum superficialis branch to the extensor carpi radialis brevis (ECRB) motor branch to restore wrist extension, and a flexor carpi radialis motor branch to posterior interosseous nerve branch to restore digital extension.[27]

There are 2 primarily theoretic benefits to nerve transfer surgery: (1) because the extensor digitorum communis (EDC) tendons are left free, there is potential for return of individual digital extension; (2) because most anterior interosseous nerve innervated motor units receive motor innervation at multiple points, there is limited loss of function of the donor motor units. Similar to other procedures that depend on regenerating nerves reaching motor endplates, however, there is a finite window during which this procedure should ideally be performed within 6 months from injury in order to allow for successful reinnervation of distal endplates in less than 12 months, although many surgeons use 12 months from injury as the procedural cutoff. In addition, patients will not notice a difference in function immediately following surgeries because functional return depends on successful regeneration of nerves to their motor endplates. This generally takes more than 6 months and may ultimately be unsuccessful, contributing to patient frustration.

Tendon transfers

Donor tendons are selected with redundant function, where tendon excursion is appropriate for their intended target, and activation during stereotyped functional activities is synergistic with the intended target. The only available functioning donor tendons are flexors. A commonly used tactic for tendon transfers is the pronator teres to the ECRB for wrist extension, the FCU to the EDC (conjoined) for digital extension, and the palmaris longus to the EPL for thumb extension.[28] However, a wide variety of alternatives and modifications exist with similarly good outcomes.

The primary benefit of tendon transfers is their early effect. Extensive physical therapy to provide guidance during a protected return to activities is generally recommended, which means there is a postoperative period of several months during which the patient will have activity restrictions and splint requirements. In addition, these tendon transfers depend on the side-to-side tenorrhaphy of the EDC tendons, sacrificing individual digital extension. However, the mechanical link between joints and powered motor units is immediately restored at the time of surgery, yielding immediate results, so patient satisfaction tends to be high.

SUMMARY

Radial nerve injuries are a common complicating factor in the treatment of humeral shaft fractures. Expectant management of nerve injury during closed treatment of fracture is standard of care. Serial physical examination of BR and ECRL function along with targeted EMGs at ~4 weeks and ~8 weeks from injury facilitates early differentiation between neuropraxic injuries (which will recover by themselves) and high-grade axonotmetic and neurontmetic injuries (which require surgical intervention). Early exploration and repair for nonrecovering injuries should be performed ~3 to 4 months from injury (earlier if there is a documented transection) using a reconstructive technique based on the size of the nerve gap. In cases whereby direct repair is unlikely to result in a good outcome, nerve transfers, tendon transfers, or a combination of both can be performed with expectation of a favorable outcome.

CLINICS CARE POINTS

- Expectant management of appropriately selected radial nerve injuries in conjunction with humeral shaft fracture requires serial examinations for early identification of nonrecovering injuries.

- Nerve transections identified during fracture fixation and not treated with acute reconstruction should be tagged under physiologic tension to prevent retraction of the nerve ends and worsening of the nerve gap, then referred for early specialist care.

- Knowledge of anatomic landmarks, including the proximal radial nerve crossing the midpoint of the humerus 2 cm proximal to the triceps aponeurosis, and the distal radial nerve crossing the lateral aspect of the humerus 10 cm proximal to the lateral epicondyle, can assist in revision nerve surgeries.

- Secondary intervention for nerve injury should be performed as early as a diagnosis of a nonrecovering nerve injury is suspected, to maximize the time for regeneration to motor endplates before loss of endplates becomes irreversible (~12 months).

DISCLOSURE

The corresponding author has a consulting agreement with DePuy Synthes.

REFERENCES

1. Ramo L, Sumrein BO, Lepola V, et al. Effect of surgery vs functional bracing on functional outcome among patients with closed displaced humeral shaft fractures: the FISH randomized clinical trial. JAMA 2020;323(18):1792–801.
2. Hendrickx LAM, Hilgersom NFJ, Alkaduhimi H, et al. Radial nerve palsy associated with closed humeral shaft fractures: a systematic review of 1758 patients. Arch Orthop Trauma Surg 2021;141(4):561–8.
3. Ekholm R, Ponzer S, Tornkvist H, et al. The Holstein-Lewis humeral shaft fracture: aspects of radial nerve injury, primary treatment, and outcome. J Orthop Trauma 2008;22(10):693–7.
4. Kong CG, Sur YJ, Jung JW, et al. Primary radial nerve palsy associated with humeral shaft fractures according to injury mechanism: is early exploration needed? J Shoulder Elbow Surg/Am Shoulder Elbow Surgeons [et al] 2021;30(12):2862–8.
5. Ring D, Chin K, Jupiter JB. Radial nerve palsy associated with high-energy humeral shaft fractures. J Hand Surg Am 2004;29(1):144–7.
6. ASSH surgical anatomy: nerve reconstruction. Chicago, IL: American Society for Surgery of the Hand; 2017.
7. Sunderland S. The anatomy and physiology of nerve injury. Muscle Nerve 1990;13(9):771–84.
8. Seddon HJ. A classification of nerve injuries. Br Med J 1942;2(4260):237–9.

9. Mackinnon SE, Dellon AL. Surgery of the peripheral nerve. New York: Thieme Medical Publishers G. Thieme Verlag; 1988.

10. Gutmann E. Factors affecting recovery of motor function after nerve lesions. J Neurol Psychiatry 1942;5(3–4):81–95.

11. Lee SK, Wolfe SW. Peripheral nerve injury and repair. J Am Acad Orthopaedic Surgeons 2000; 8(4):243–52.

12. Shao YC, Harwood P, Grotz MR, et al. Radial nerve palsy associated with fractures of the shaft of the humerus: a systematic review. J Bone Joint Surg Br 2005;87(12):1647–52.

13. Ostermann RC, Lang NW, Joestl J, et al. Fractures of the humeral shaft with primary radial nerve palsy: do injury mechanism, fracture type, or treatment influence nerve recovery? J Clin Med 2019; 8(11).

14. Abrams RA, Ziets RJ, Lieber RL, et al. Anatomy of the radial nerve motor branches in the forearm. J Hand Surg Am 1997;22(2):232–7.

15. Aminoff MJ. Electrophysiologic testing for the diagnosis of peripheral nerve injuries. Anesthesiology 2004;100(5):1298–303.

16. Oh SJ. Electromyographic studies in peripheral nerve injuries. South Med J 1976;69(2):177–82.

17. Yang KH, Han DY, Kim HJ. Intramedullary entrapment of the radial nerve associated with humeral shaft fracture. J Orthop Trauma 1997;11(3):224–6.

18. Mackinnon S. Grabb and Smith's plastic surgery - chapter 9 principles and techniques of peripheral nerve repair, grafts, and transfers. 7th edition ed. Philadelphia: Wolters Kluwer/Lippincott Williams & Wilkins Health; 2014.

19. Moore AM, Wagner IJ, Fox IK. Principles of nerve repair in complex wounds of the upper extremity. Semin Plast Surg 2015;29(1):40–7.

20. Tupper JW, Crick JC, Matteck LR. Fascicular nerve repairs. A comparative study of epineurial and fascicular (perineurial) techniques. Orthop Clin North America 1988;19(1):57–69.

21. Wang E, Inaba K, Byerly S, et al. Optimal timing for repair of peripheral nerve injuries. J Trauma Acute Care Surg 2017;83(5):875–81.

22. Zlotolow DA, Catalano LW 3rd, Barron OA, et al. Surgical exposures of the humerus. J Am Acad Orthopaedic Surgeons 2006;14(13):754–65.

23. Kornfeld T, Vogt PM, Radtke C. Nerve grafting for peripheral nerve injuries with extended defect sizes. Wien Med Wochenschr 2019;169(9–10):240–51.

24. Compton J, Owens J, Day M, et al. Systematic review of tendon transfer versus nerve transfer for the restoration of wrist extension in isolated traumatic radial nerve palsy. J Am Acad Orthop Surg Glob Res Rev 2018;2(4):e001.

25. Patterson JMM, Russo SA, El-Haj M, et al. Radial nerve palsy: nerve transfer versus tendon transfer to restore function. Hand (N Y) 2021. 1558944720988126.

26. Bertelli JA. Nerve versus tendon transfer for radial nerve paralysis reconstruction. J Hand Surg Am 2020;45(5):418–26.

27. Davidge KM, Yee A, Kahn LC, et al. Median to radial nerve transfers for restoration of wrist, finger, and thumb extension. J Hand Surg Am 2013;38(9): 1812–27.

28. Sammer DM, Chung KC. Tendon transfers: part I. Principles of transfer and transfers for radial nerve palsy. Plast Reconstr Surg 2009;123(5):169e–77e.

Peripheral Nerve Management in Extremity Amputations

John T. Richards, MD[a,b,*], Michael D. Baird, MD[a,1],
Scott M. Tintle, MD[a,1], Jason M. Souza, MD[c],
Christopher H. Renninger, MD[a,b,1],
Benjamin K. Potter, MD[a,1]

KEYWORDS

- Amputation • Neuroma • Phantom limb pain • Nerve injury • Targeted muscle reinnervation
- Regenerative peripheral nerve interface

KEY POINTS

- Many amputees will deal with neuroma pain or phantom limb pain at some point in their postoperative course.
- The thoughtful surgical management of major peripheral nerves in the setting of extremity amputation improves outcomes for amputees, decreasing the risk of reoperation and maximizing prosthetic use.
- Targeted muscle reinnervation (TMR) and regenerative peripheral nerve interface (RPNI) creation have emerged as advanced alternatives to previous techniques, such as traction neurectomy, with promising clinical outcomes.
- While TMR and RPNI can be successful in managing symptomatic neuroma and phantom limb pain, performing these techniques acutely, at the time of primary amputation, may prevent them from developing altogether.

INTRODUCTION

The effective management of major peripheral nerves in the setting of extremity amputation is critical to maximizing patient function and clinical outcomes. Up to 80% of amputees will experience a complication of some kind during their treatment, nearly half of which are due to nerve-related pain.[1] In addition, up to 50% of amputees live with some degree of chronic pain, which is often attributed to symptomatic neuromata and/or phantom limb pain.[2] This disability is associated with the need for reoperation, the risk for opioid dependence, decreased mobility, and decreased quality of life. Thirty percent of amputees who discontinue prosthetic use cite symptomatic neuroma pain as the principal factor.[3] While increasingly recognized

[a] Department of Orthopaedic Surgery, Uniformed Services University-Walter Reed Department of Surgery, Walter Reed National Military Medical Center, Bethesda, MD, USA; [b] Department of Orthopaedics, R Adams Cowley Shock Trauma Center, University of Maryland School of Medicine, Baltimore, MD, USA; [c] Department of Plastic and Reconstructive Surgery, The Ohio State University Wexner Medical Center, Columbus, OH, USA

[1] The designated authors are employees of the U.S. Government. This work was prepared as part of their official duties. Title 17 U.S C.§105 provides that "Copyright protection under this title is not available for any work of the United States Government." Title 17 U.S C. §101 defined a U.S. Government work as a work prepared by a military service member or employees of the U.S. Government as part of that person's official duties. The opinions or assertions contained in this article are the private views of the authors and are not to be construed as reflecting the views, policy, or positions of the Department of the Navy, Department of the Army, Department of Defense, nor the U.S. Government.

* Corresponding author. 22 S. Greene Street, Baltimore, MD 21201.
E-mail address: john.richards@som.umaryland.edu

Orthop Clin N Am 53 (2022) 155–166
https://doi.org/10.1016/j.ocl.2022.01.002
0030-5898/22/© 2022 Elsevier Inc. All rights reserved.

today, nerve-related amputation pain is not a new problem. In 1829, William Wood provided one of the first case series and his experience on the treatment of neuromas.[4] More recently, there has been renewed interest in the treatment of symptomatic neuromata and phantom pain in the amputee. In the first decade of the conflicts in Iraq and Afghanistan, over 1000 U.S. military service members sustained at least one major extremity amputation.[5,6] Recognition of this trend led the United States Department of Defense to fund major research initiatives to address this increasingly appreciated problem, reinvigorating efforts to improve outcomes in this population.[5,6] Nonetheless, neuroma pain and phantom limb pain in amputees is far from isolated to military personnel. In the United States, there are more than 185,000 amputations performed per year and by the year 2050, there will be an estimated 3.6 million people living with an amputation.[2,6–8] Both preemptive and delayed surgical management of peripheral nerves in the setting of major amputation improves symptomatic neuroma and phantom limb pain.[9] While treatment strategies exist to manage the sequela of nerve-related pain, the authors believe that many of these complications can be prevented with a thoughtful approach from the primary amputation. We present a review of the current state of the art in the management of peripheral nerves in the setting of major extremity amputation.

Background

Nerve-related pain in the setting of extremity amputation is one of the many causes of residual limb pain and is often subclassified into neuroma-related pain and phantom limb pain. Neuroma pain is that which is attributable to the formation of symptomatic neuroma. A neuroma is a disorganized collection of axons, Schwann cells, and connective tissue that results as a sequela of a transected peripheral nerve (Fig. 1). When a peripheral nerve is transected

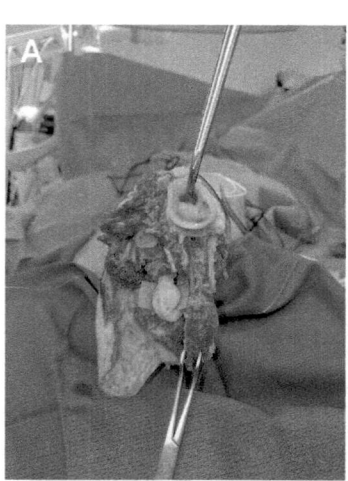
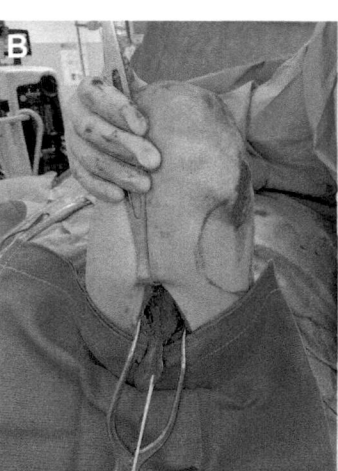
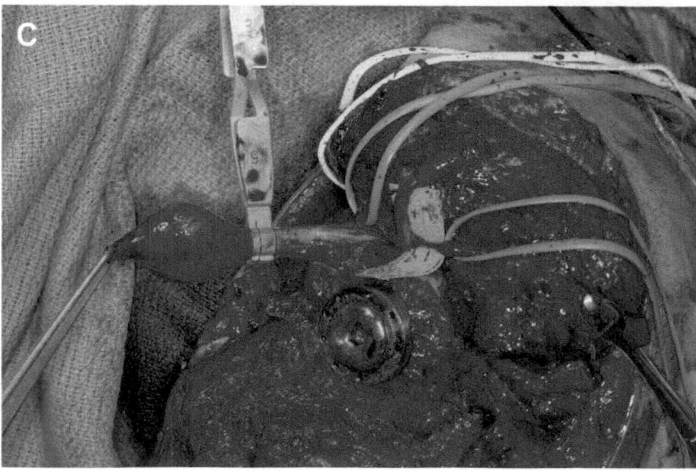

Fig. 1. Examples of multiple neuromata at the time of surgery. (A) A tibial neuroma in the setting of transtibial amputation (B) A sciatic neuroma in the setting of transfemoral amputation (C) A Median neuroma in the setting of stage I osseointegration for transhumeral amputation before TMR. The blue vessel loop denotes the target and yellow is the donor nerve.

such as in the setting of amputation, the distal portion of the nerve undergoes the process of Wallerian degeneration. This coordinated process is facilitated by macrophages and inflammatory cells and prepares the distal nerve to facilitate regeneration.[10–12] As the distal nerve degenerates, Schwann cells form into an organized scaffold and along with other glial cells produce cytokines and neurotrophic factors promoting proximal axonal regeneration.[10,12,13] The proximal portions of the cut axons begin sprouting as early as 3 days following an injury.[10,12] Guided by neurotrophic factors, these sprouting axons can grow into endoneurial tubes and ultimately reinnervate their end organ. In the setting of a standard amputation, there is no distal regulation of proximal nerve regeneration. Without a scaffold for growth, neurotrophic factors to guide them, or a distal target to (re)innervate, the unregulated growth of the proximal nerve produces a collection of disordered axons, Schwann cells, and connective tissue known as a neuroma. This disordered and dysfunctional neural tissue often becomes hyper-excitable with spontaneous ectopic activity or excitation with minimal stimuli such as light touch or direct pressure. This activity is thought to be due to disordered regulation of transduction molecules, aberrant neural connections, and dysfunction of sodium and potassium channels.[3] For amputees, neuromata result in painful and often radiating symptoms due to mild, or even in the absence of, external stimuli. While not always symptomatic, the sheer number of nerves affected after amputation and the superficial location of many major peripheral nerves make them prone to producing symptoms, most notably with prosthetic use.[6] These symptomatic neuromata can be debilitating for amputees, creating pain, limiting the use of socket-based prosthetics, and ultimately limiting mobility and quality of life.

Phantom limb pain refers to the perception of pain in the missing limb such as sensing pain in the foot in the setting of a transtibial amputation. Phantom pain is a distinct subcategory of phantom limb sensation, which refers to any sensation perceived within the missing limb including hyperpathia or paresthesias. Phantom sensation in the absence of phantom pain is rarely bothersome and often perceived as an asset by persons with limb loss.[9] The presentation and quality of phantom limb pain are variable, but patients most commonly describe throbbing, burning, and/or clenching, among other sensations. Phantom limb pain is separate from the more focal pain associated with

neuroma; however, the 2 are thought to be related to one another. The concept of sensation within a missing limb in the setting of amputation was first reported by Ambrose Pare, a French military surgeon.[14] An American Civil War surgeon, Silas Weir Mitchell, later described the term "phantom limb pain" and wrote on his experience treating soldiers on the battlefield.[14,15] The exact mechanism of phantom limb sensation and pain remains unknown but is thought to be multifactorial, with a combination of peripheral and central factors including abnormal signaling from injured afferent nerve fibers and eventually changes within the cortical gray matter.[7,16–18] New data suggest a complex interplay between the central and peripheral nervous system whereby disordered hyperactivity associated with symptomatic neuroma leads to the dysregulation of excitatory and inhibitory processes in the central nervous system known as central sensitization.[3] Much like neuroma pain, there is a broad range in the reported incidence of phantom limb pain, ranging from 25% to 79%[7,14,19–22] Risk factors associated with increased phantom limb pain include female sex, upper extremity amputation, traumatic amputation, depression and other psychiatric illness, and pre-existing pain in the amputated extremity.[7,9,14] The onset of phantom limb pain can be immediate or delayed months or years and, while it has been shown to often decrease with time, eventual spontaneous resolution is far from guaranteed.[23,24]

Patient Evaluation
Amputation may be indicated to treat a diverse array of clinical circumstances including trauma, oncologic, vascular, or congenital conditions. Patients may present with the need for an elective amputation or with nerve-related pain complaints associated with an existing amputation. The initial evaluation of any patient should consist of a thorough history and physical examination detailing the need for or reason for amputation, current symptoms, and any previous surgical history relevant to the extremity in question. It is important to assess for a history of psychiatric illness, pre-existing chronic pain, and other risk factors for chronic pain. In patients with an existing amputation presenting with pain, the history should focus on the quality and location of the pain, aggravating and alleviating factors, prosthetic type and the amount of use, mobility goals, and any previous treatments. The patient should further be evaluated for comorbid conditions such as chronic pain, low back pain, or spine pathology.

Physical examination is critical to evaluate the neurologic function of the affected limb including a detailed motor and sensory examination. It is important to note any previous surgical incisions, the character, and quality of the skin and soft tissue envelope, along the shape contour of the underlying bone. Special attention should be paid to areas of tenderness on palpation and any provocative symptoms such as a Tinel's sign. A Tinel's sign, or shockwave-like symptoms with palpation or percussion along the course of a major peripheral nerve, should raise suspicion for symptomatic neuroma, particularly if the patient confirms that this clinical stimulation replicates their symptoms. While nerve-related pain in the setting of amputation is common, it is important to identify and treat other causes of residual limb pain such as infection, bony prominences, inadequate padding, poor skin quality, or excessive mobility of the soft tissue envelope. These often occur concomitantly and can be addressed during the same surgical intervention.

Radiographs are routinely obtained to assess the osseous anatomy and evaluate for any heterotopic bone or radiopaque foreign bodies. Ultrasound can be useful for identifying and visualizing the location of neuromata. However, it is important to note that nearly all amputees will have identifiable neuromata of some size and that not all of these are necessarily symptomatic; that is, the presence of a neuroma(s) is not in and of itself an indication for surgery or even additional treatment. Advanced imaging such as CT scan or MRI scan may be indicated in certain cases; however, the authors do not find them to be routinely necessary. It is important to remember that fluid collections are prevalent in this patient population and nearly always benign.[25] Unless there is other clinical evidence of infection on history or physical examination, identification of a fluid collection in the amputee should not delay treatment or lead to further unnecessary workup.

While common, neuroma pain in amputees can often either remain unidentified or misdiagnosed, leading to failed revision surgical intervention and poor outcomes. In the setting of revision operative management for amputees presenting with pain in their residual limb, neuroma-related pain should be considered in the differential diagnosis because of complex clinical presentations. Finding a clear etiology for postamputation pain may require attempts at multiple nonsurgical treatments such as prosthetic modification and interventional diagnostics. A multidisciplinary approach to these patients helps to achieve the best possible outcome with coordination and close communication between surgeons, pain management specialists, psychiatrists, physiatrists, prosthetists, and occupational and physical therapists. Finally, as with any consideration for revision surgery, the treatment team should endeavor to identify a clear diagnosis and a clear treatment goal before proceeding with any surgical intervention.

Nonsurgical Treatment Options

The treatment of extremity pain for amputees is often broken down into 3 categories: pharmacologic, psychological, and physical.[1,7] The primary pharmacologic interventions for nerve-related extremity pain in the amputee are consistent with standard pain treatments, consisting of nonsteroidal anti-inflammatories (NSAIDs), acetaminophen, narcotics, antidepressants, anticonvulsants, nerve modulators, nerve blocks, and local anesthetic patches.[1,26] Targeted steroid injections combined with local anesthetic can provide therapeutic pain relief and valuable diagnostic feedback which can help delineate the primary pain sources in the residual limb. Some component of phantom limb and residual limb pain is thought to be related to hyperactivity of N-methyl D-aspartate (NMDA) receptors. Small series have shown the efficacy of sedative-hypnotics such as ketamine given in bolus, which may reset components of this pathway and improve phantom limb sensation and nerve-related residual limb pain.[27] Other medications that modulate the NMDA pathway remain a promising area of future research for nonoperative treatment.

The primary psychological treatments for the treatment of phantom limb and nerve-related residual limb pain include mirror therapy, cognitive behavioral therapy, and desensitization therapy. Mirror therapy, effective primarily for phantom limb sensations, uses the patient's intact contralateral limb with well-positioned mirrors and provides visual feedback to the brain, effectively tricking the brain into "seeing" the missing limb.[28] Nonoperative physical treatments of amputation pain include transcutaneous electrical nerve stimulation (TENS), spinal cord stimulators, nerve ablation, ultrasound therapy, physical and occupational rehabilitation, exercise, and massage.[1]

Surgical Treatment Options

Before the development of more modern strategies, a myriad of techniques has been described for the treatment and prevention of postamputation neuroma. There are more than 150 reported surgical techniques described for the treatment of symptomatic neuroma.[6] As with other disciplines of surgery, the sheer number of techniques described suggests that none demonstrated superior efficacy. However, meta-analysis data suggest that surgical intervention is superior to nonoperative management with 75% of patients gaining improvement from surgery.[29]

One of the simplest forms of neuroma treatment is simple resection or traction neurectomy. This technique is popular, especially during primary amputation, due to its ease and speed. The goal of the technique is to traction the distal end of the affected nerve and transects it more proximally, causing it to retract into a more proximal, often deeper, and putatively less symptomatic location. While it is widely performed, this technique has consistently demonstrated inferior outcomes when compared with other treatments.[30] Numerous other techniques have been described with varying levels of success. These techniques are aimed at either burying the involved nerve in a less symptomatic location or capping it to prevent or contain sprouting axons and subsequent neuroma formation.[31]

Several techniques describe the transposition of the terminal nerve end into various target tissues, including vein, bone, and muscle. Implantation of nerves into veins has been described with success in animal models; however, there is very limited evidence exists regarding efficacy in human subjects.[32,33] Technical difficulties such as the nerve withdrawing from the vein and subsequently reforming the neuroma have also been noted.[34] Transposition into bone has also been described with modest outcomes, though one recent case report notes that fracture is a risk specific to this method.[35,36] Transposition into muscle is one of the most commonly described techniques, with "simple" transposition into muscle described as having over an 80% success rate in several small series.[37] While the goal of these techniques is often described as placing the nerve in a less symptomatic location, the recipient tissue bed ultimately remains innervated. Without "a place to go or something to do," the implanted peripheral nerve will still be at risk to sprout new axons and produce a subsequent, potentially symptomatic, neuroma.

As opposed to transposing the nerve to a less symptomatic location, other techniques aim to cap the proximal end of the transected nerve to prevent the regrowth of the sprouting axons. Numerous autogenous and synthetic materials have been described to include synthetic resins, silicone, free vascular graft, and most recently with acellular nerve allograft.[38–41] None of these techniques has shown reproducible outcomes in clinical practice. Other described techniques involve suturing free peripheral nerve ends together. Centro-central anastomosis, whereby 2 nerve ends are brought together, and end-to-side neurorrhaphy, whereby an epineurial window is made and the transected nerve is implanted, have both been studied in humans and animals. These techniques have also failed to gain widespread adoption due to failure to demonstrate reproducible outcomes when evaluated in larger studies and are thought to be limited due to their technical difficulty.[31,42–44] In our experience treating patients with persistent symptoms who had undergone the procedure elsewhere, centro-central anastomosis tends to result in the formation of a very large, combined or composite, neuroma and is not effective.

Regenerative Peripheral Nerve Interface

Regenerative peripheral nerve interface (RPNI) is a technique where a small piece of devascularized, denervated muscle tissue is transferred to the affected nerve (Fig. 2). RPNI improves on the basis of previous techniques by not just placing the nerve into a less symptomatic location but providing the affected nerve a denervated tissue to reinnervate.[45] Because the nerve now has a target, it is hypothesized that fewer disorganized axons exist to create symptomatic neuroma.[46] The basis of RPNI was initially to amplify targets and improve transduction for myoelectric prosthetics using implanted electrodes.[47,48] Myoelectric prosthetics are externally powered devices that sense proximal muscle contraction and translate this to the volitional movement of the prosthetic. Following RPNI, subsequent histologic studies noted the decreased formation of disorganized axon growth and neuroma formation prompting clinical investigations into its use for neuroma prevention.[45,49–51] The reduction in neuropathic pain and phantom limb pain is hypothesized to also be related to the nerve now having a target, reducing ectopic signals, and decreasing the phenomenon of central sensitization.[3,52]

REGENERATIVE PERIPHERAL NERVE INTERFACE

Surgical Technique

Multiple descriptions of the surgical technique have been published.[3] In general, an approximately 3 cm × 2 cm x 0.5 cm free muscle graft is used. It is important to avoid placing too large of graft as this can interfere with perfusion of the

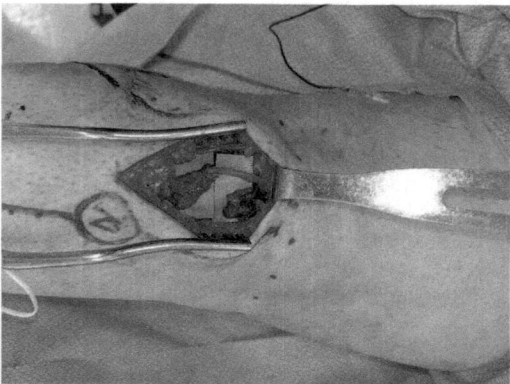

Fig. 2. Clinical photo of RPNI. The sural nerve has been wrapped with a free muscle graft according to the RPNI technique described to address a sural neuroma following a transtibial amputation.

muscle from the wound bed and lead to greater necrosis. The desired peripheral nerve is then placed within the muscle graft, ideally parallel to the direction of the muscle fibers. The epineurium is sewn into the free muscle tissue with a small (5–0 or 6–0) suture. The muscle is then wrapped around the nerve and sewn to itself with absorbable suture. Following implantation, the denervated muscle tissue provides a target for the sprouting axons from the regenerating nerve to reinnervate. While concerns exist over placing devitalized tissue into a wound bed, studies demonstrate the muscle tissue is initially supported via imbibition and, following re-innervation, is eventually re-vascularized via vasa nervorum and the adjacent soft tissues.[53] In the setting of a large peripheral nerve, such as the sciatic nerve, multiple grafts (often 3–4) can be utilized to avoid discordance between the number of nerve fascicles and target motor or sensory endplates.

While it is logical that efferent motor nerves in a transected peripheral nerve would feasibly reinnervate free muscle tissue, it is less clear with afferent sensory axons. While the exact mechanism is still under investigation, multiple studies have shown promising results with decreased neuroma formation even in isolated sensory nerves.[3] Histologic and immunohistochemical analysis of sensory nerves implanted in denervated skeletal muscle demonstrated little evidence of neuroma in a rat model. While it is unlikely the sensory nerves will reinnervate the muscle to provide a functional motor unit for myoelectric control, the basis for sensory nerves to provide the trophic stabilization of devitalized skeletal muscle is well established.[54,55] Additionally, it is thought that the sensory end organs, such as Golgi tendon organs and spindle cells, provide viable targets for these sensory afferents, which is supported by animal models.[56]

Regenerative Peripheral Nerve Interface Outcomes

The clinical outcomes of RPNI have been optimistic. The retrospective study by Woo and colleagues demonstrated 73% of patients with a significant reduction in neuroma pain and 53% with decreased phantom pain along with uniformly high patient satisfaction. More recent studies have shown it to be as effective in managing neuroma in the upper extremity including isolated sensory, digital neuromas.[45] Most recently, Kubiak and colleagues produced a retrospective study showing that prophylactic RPNI at the time of primary amputation could result in a significant decrease in phantom pain and a potential decrease in the incidence of neuroma formation.[57] None of the 45 patients who underwent RPNI developed symptomatic neuroma compared with 6/45 (13%) in the control group. Additionally, only 51% of patients who underwent RPNI reported phantom limb pain compared with 91% in the control group.

Targeted Muscle Reinnervation

Like RPNI, targeted muscle reinnervation (TMR) is a surgical technique that aims to provide reinnervation to otherwise unutilized peripheral nerves. TMR is distinct from RPNI in that instead of transferring these unutilized peripheral nerves to the devitalized muscle, it instead aims to transfer them to expendable, intact motor units (Fig. 3). Like RPNI, TMR was initially developed to amplify the number of motor unit targets for myoelectric control in the setting of proximal amputations.[58] The basis for the development of TMR was that for proximal amputations there are too few voluntary, motor unit targets to allow for the number of desired prosthetic motions, such as hand opening and closing. However, the proximal portions of major peripheral nerves which innervate the distal extremity and control these functions remain unutilized in a standard amputation. TMR uses these transected nerves to reinnervate a motor unit(s) of a more proximal muscle group and provide additional targets, to serve as a biologic amplifier for intuitive myoelectric control and further giving these otherwise unexploited nerves "somewhere to go and something to do." Its benefit in the management of nerve pain was noted after subsequent clinical studies found that patients treated with TMR suffered from less

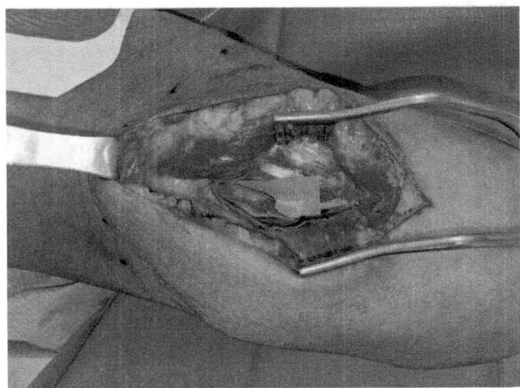

Fig. 3. Clinical photo of TMR. The common peroneal nerve has been coapted to the motor branch to the lateral gastrocnemius muscle to treat a common peroneal neuroma after transtibial amputation.

symptomatic neuroma and improved phantom limb pain.[6,59–64] In a rabbit neuroma model, TMR reduced sprouting, decreased myelinated fiber counts, and increased the myelinated fibers size of the transferred nerves bringing them back to a more normal preinjury state.[65] In addition to its prosthesis control advantages, repurposing these nerves decreases the formation of symptomatic neuroma and phantom limb pain in the residual limb.

TARGETED MUSCLE REINNERVATION
Surgical Technique
The general technique for TMR involves the identification and primary coaptation of a discrete, previously intact, and functional motor nerve to the terminal end of a transected peripheral nerve. This can be performed in the setting of primary amputation or as a subsequent revision procedure in the setting of an existing amputation. TMR in the acute setting has multiple perceived benefits. The surgical dissection is technically easier as virgin anatomic planes are providing improved the access and identification of key structures. In addition to less scar formation associated with dissection, acute TMR provides a more ideal neurophysiologic environment for healing the transferred nerves.[64,65]

The specific motor targets for major peripheral nerves for common upper and lower extremity amputation levels are well described in the literature and outlined in Table 1.[60,63,66–68] In general, loupe magnification is preferred for this procedure to facilitate proper visualization. The donor motor branch is identified with the use of a nerve stimulator. The motor nerve target is transected approximately 1 cm from its recipient muscle belly to facilitate rapid reinnervation. Performing the coaptation close to the motor entry point allows for burial of the coaptation site within the newly denervated muscle target, thus providing a receptive environment for sprouting axons that are not directly coapted end-to-end to the recipient's nerve due to a size mismatch with the larger donor nerve. The coaptation to the recipient motor branch is most frequently performed with a single centralizing 8 to 0 suture, which is then reinforced with 2 or 3 additional 6 to 0 epineurial to empymisial sutures. Alternatively, a large size discrepancy between the donor nerve and recipient nerve can be addressed by splitting the donor nerve into fascicular components and individually coapting these fascicles to different target motor branches (typically of the same muscle, which we have termed "split TMR"), if available. We recommend avoiding excessive epineurial sutures to compensate for a significant size mismatch, as the foreign suture material can impair healing. Fibrin glue can be applied to further protect the coaptation site.

Optimal muscle targets are those that have lost their insertion site following amputation and are effectively no longer functional or those which have multiple redundant muscle bellies. If possible, the motor branch should be close to the desired donor nerve to prevent significant undue tension. If performed for myoelectric control, superficial muscles are preferable. Additionally, excision of the distal neuroma is often performed as a matter of course, but is not required and not recommended if additional extensive dissection and time are required.[60]

TARGETED MUSCLE REINNERVATION OUTCOMES

Multiple authors have reported favorable outcomes with the use of TMR for the treatment and prevention of symptomatic neuroma and phantom limb pain.[6,22,59,61,62] Souza and colleagues reported one of the first retrospective series of 26 patients who underwent upper extremity TMR. While the primary motivation for TMR in these patients was prosthetic control, none of these patients developed new neuroma-related pain in the postoperative period. In addition, 14 of the 15 patients who presented with neuroma pain had complete resolution of their symptoms.[6]

Frantz and colleagues prospectively studied TMR in the setting of primary amputation and found low rates of phantom limb pain and 85% of lower extremity amputees reporting meaningful prosthetic use.[22] Dumanian and colleagues

Table 1
The authors' typical management of major extremity nerves in the setting of upper and lower extremity amputations by common amputation level

Amputation Level	Nerve	Typical or Preferred Option	Additional Options
Transradial	Median	Flexor digitorum superficialis Flexor digitorum profundus	
	Ulnar	Flexor carpi ulnaris	Flexor pollicis longus
	Superficial branch Radial	Extensor carpi radialis longus or brevis	Flexor digitorum profundus
	Lateral antebrachial cutaneous (LABC)	RPNI	
	Medial antebrachial cutaneous (MABC)	RPNI	
Transhumeral	Median	Short head of biceps brachii	
	Ulnar	Brachialis	
	Radial	Lateral head triceps	
	Medial antebrachial cutaneous	RPNI	
	Lateral antebrachial cutaneous	RPNI	
Transtibial	Superficial peroneal	Peroneus longus or brevis	
	Deep peroneal	Tibialis anterior	Peroneus longus or brevis, medial soleus
	Tibial	Medial or lateral gastrocnemius	Tibialis posterior, soleus
	Sural	RPNI	Tibialis posterior, soleus
	Saphenous	RPNI	Medial gastrocnemius, medial soleus, vastus medialis
Transfemoral	Common peroneal	Biceps femoris	Semimembranosus, semitendinosus
	Tibial	Semimembranosus	Biceps femoris, semitendinosus
	Saphenous	RPNI	
	Posterior cutaneous nerve thigh	RPNI	

1. RPNI remains an option for any nerve when TMR is not possible or unfeasible
2. Options for transhumeral and transfemoral can be generalized to elbow disarticulation and knee disarticulation, respectively
3. Shoulder and hip disarticulation levels not described here as the proximal nature of the amputations make standard transfers unpredictable with significant variation between cases

performed the first prospective randomized, controlled trial for the treatment of symptomatic neuroma in amputees. The investigators randomized 28 patients to TMR or neuroma resection and implantation into a muscle with results favoring improved outcomes in the TMR group.[59] Residual limb pain and phantom limb pain were decreased in the TMR group. Valerio and colleagues reported the results of a multicenter cohort evaluating TMR at the time of primary amputation for the preemptive treatment of neuroma and phantom limb pain.[1] Fifty-one patients undergoing major limb amputation with immediate TMR were compared with a cohort of 438 amputees who had previously undergone standard amputation without TMR. The TMR group was 3.03 times less likely to have phantom limb pain and nearly 4 times less likely to have residual limb pain. Patients who underwent TMR had a 4-point decrease in NRS scores compared with the control group (MCID 2 points) and significantly decreased opioid use.

TARGETED MUSCLE REINNERVATION VERSUS REGENERATIVE PERIPHERAL NERVE INTERFACE

To date, there are no clinical studies directly comparing TMR to RPNI. However, there are several important similarities and differences between the 2 techniques. Both TMR and RPNI are novel surgical techniques aimed at treating and preventing neuroma formation, and both offer potential advantages for myoelectric prosthesis control. TMR further can be used toward this end with commercially available interfaces, whereas RPNI remains experimental in this regard. The 2 techniques work by providing a transected peripheral nerve a target of denervated muscle for reinnervation. One clear difference between the techniques is that TMR requires the presence and sacrifice of intact motor units. For TMR to be considered a viable treatment option, the patient must have intact functional motor units that can be sacrificed. This can be complicated in proximal amputations with fewer targets or in the setting of more proximal or incomplete nerve injuries. Furthermore, there is a theoretic risk of weakness associated with the denervation of intact motor units; however, the clinical significance of this is uncertain and the most common motor nerve-muscle targets used have no meaningful residual function due to the absence of the distal joint. In contrast, RPNI uses devitalized muscle, which is often abundant, and discarded at the time of primary amputation. Even in the setting of an existing amputation, the harvest of small muscle grafts for RPNI provides minimal morbidity to the patient.

Another clear distinction between the 2 techniques is that TMR is significantly more labor-intensive and technically demanding. TMR often requires significantly more equipment and operating room support than RPNI, with specific instruments such as loupe magnification,

microsurgical instruments, and a nerve stimulator. Additionally, the procedure often requires significantly more dissection to facilitate exposure of motor unit targets and thus also takes longer. In contrast, RPNI requires less time, less surgical dissection, and can be accomplished with minimal microsurgical experience. However, RPNI does leave de-vascularized tissue within the residual limb, as previously noted, and the muscle reinnervation targets are both smaller initially and prone to further necrosis and contraction before revascularization and healing. Further, RPNI typically does not provide a motor nerve conduit for reinnervation but instead relies on spontaneous and unorganized axonal sprouting into the denervated muscle graft.

COMPLICATIONS

The complications associated with TMR, RPNI, and other surgical treatments for nerve-related amputation pain are few, with the primary risk being treatment failure. With both TMR and RPNI, there is a risk of failure of reinnervation with likely resultant neuroma reformation. While the failure of reinnervation may not always result in clinical symptoms, in the case of TMR, the loss of the motor unit could result in mild weakness along with loss of a myoelectric target. One risk for treatment failure specific to TMR is due to the risk of reinnervation of the denervated motor unit by the native motor branch that is transected at the time of surgery.[60] This risk can be mitigated with segmental resection of the motor nerve to the muscle unit being used.

SUMMARY AND FUTURE DIRECTIONS

It is the authors' strong belief that a thoughtful approach to the management of major peripheral nerves at the time of primary amputation decreases postamputation neuroma and phantom limb pain, improves prosthetic use, decreases reoperation, and ultimately improves outcomes for amputees. Modern surgical techniques such as TMR and RPNI have emerged as exciting alternatives to traditional neuroma prevention strategies which primarily aimed to place the inevitable neuroma in a less symptomatic location. TMR and RPNI have shown promising results for the treatment and prevention of symptomatic neuroma and phantom limb pain by providing denervated muscle targets for reinnervation. While there are distinct differences and advantages between each of these techniques, they are often used together for optimal effect. Recent studies have even described hybrid procedures which harness the theoretic advantages of both techniques.[52] In addition to the treatment of postamputation pain, both techniques have the added benefit of improved myoelectric control. Despite all the recent advances, there is still enormous potential for further research. Future studies will provide larger, comparative outcome data for both TMR and RPNI determine the ideal indications for each technique along with harnessing their full potential for prosthetic control.

CLINICS CARE POINTS

- Postamputation neuroma pain and phantom limb pain are prevalent among amputees resulting in chronic pain, poor tolerance of prosthetics, and the need for reoperation.
- The formation of neuromas following the transection of major peripheral nerves in the setting of extremity amputation is predictable and related to the complex phenomenon of phantom limb pain through peripheral and central factors.
- The optimal treatment of nerve-related amputation pain requires the coordination and close communication of a multidisciplinary team including surgeons, pain management specialists, psychiatrists, physiatrists, prosthetists, and occupational and physical therapists.
- While nonsurgical strategies have a role, the surgical management of postamputation neuroma pain and phantom limb pain is effective for patients who fail conservative treatment.
- TMR and RPNI are exciting new surgical techniques which treat and prevent nerve-related amputation pain by providing major peripheral nerves denervated muscle tissue for reinnervation. These techniques provide these otherwise unutilized nerves with "somewhere to go and something to do," resulting in decreased nerve-related pain and improved possibilities for myoelectric prosthetics.

DISCLOSURE

All authors report no disclosures or conflict of interest.

REFERENCES

1. Ducic I, Mesbahi AN, Attinger CE, et al. The role of peripheral nerve surgery in the treatment of chronic pain associated with amputation stumps. Plast Reconstr Surg 2008;121(3):908–14.
2. Peters BR, Russo SA, West JM, et al. Targeted muscle reinnervation for the management of pain in the setting of major limb amputation. Sage Open Med 2020;8. https://doi.org/10.1177/2050312120959180. 2050312120959180.
3. Santosa KB, Oliver JD, Cederna PS, et al. Regenerative peripheral nerve interfaces for prevention and management of neuromas. Clin Plast Surg 2020; 47(2):311–21.
4. Wood W. Observations on neuroma, with cases and histories of the disease. Trans Med Chir Soc Edinb 1829;3(Pt 2):367–433.
5. Stansbury LG, Lalliss SJ, Branstetter JG, et al. Amputations in U.S. Military Personnel in the Current Conflicts in Afghanistan and Iraq. J Orthop Trauma 2008;22(1):43–6.
6. Souza JM, Cheesborough JE, Ko JH, et al. Targeted muscle reinnervation: a novel approach to postamputation neuroma pain. Clin Orthop Relat Res 2014;472(10):2984–90.
7. Bowen JB, Wee CE, Kalik J, et al. Targeted muscle reinnervation to improve pain, prosthetic tolerance, and bioprosthetic outcomes in the amputee. Adv Wound Care 2017;6(8):261–7.
8. Ziegler-Graham K, MacKenzie EJ, Ephraim PL, et al. Estimating the prevalence of limb loss in the United States: 2005 to 2050. Arch Phys Med Rehabil 2008; 89(3):422–9.
9. Prantl L, Schreml S, Heine N, et al. Surgical treatment of chronic phantom limb sensation and limb pain after lower limb amputation. Plast Reconstr Surg 2006;118(7):1562–72.
10. Oliveira KMC, Pindur L, Han Z, et al. Time course of traumatic neuroma development. PLoS One 2018; 13(7):e0200548. https://doi.org/10.1371/journal. pone.0200548.
11. Namgung U. The role of schwann cell-axon interaction in peripheral nerve regeneration. Cells Tissues Organs 2015;200(1):6–12.
12. Wood MD, Mackinnon SE. Pathways regulating modality-specific axonal regeneration in peripheral nerve. Exp Neurol 2015;265:171–5.
13. Stoll G, Müller HW. Nerve injury, axonal degeneration and neural regeneration: basic insights. Brain Pathol 1999;9(2):313–25.
14. Subedi B, Grossberg GT. Phantom limb pain: mechanisms and treatment approaches. Pain Res Treat 2011;2011:864605.
15. Louis ED, York GK. Weir Mitchell's observations on sensory localization and their influence on Jacksonian neurology. Neurology 2006;66(8): 1241–4.
16. Bolognini N, Olgiati E, Maravita A, et al. Motor and parietal cortex stimulation for phantom limb pain and sensations. Pain 2013;154(8):1274–80.

17. Elbert T, Rockstroh B. Reorganization of Human Cerebral Cortex: The Range of Changes Following Use and Injury. Neurosci 2004;10(2):129–41.

18. Preißler S, Feiler J, Dietrich C, et al. Gray matter changes following limb amputation with high and low intensities of phantom limb pain. Cereb Cortex 2013;23(5):1038–48.

19. Richardson C, Glenn S, Nurmikko T, et al. Incidence of phantom phenomena including phantom limb pain 6 months after major lower limb amputation in patients with peripheral vascular disease. Clin J Pain 2006;22(4):353–8.

20. Schley MT, Wilms P, Toepfner S, et al. Painful and Nonpainful Phantom and Stump Sensations in Acute Traumatic Amputees. J Trauma Inj Infect Crit Care 2008;65(4):858–64.

21. Reiber GE, McFarland LV, Hubbard S, et al. Service-members and veterans with major traumatic limb loss from Vietnam war and OIF/OEF conflicts: survey methods, participants, and summary findings. J Rehabil Res Dev 2010;47(4):275.

22. Frantz TL, Everhart JS, West JM, et al. Targeted muscle reinnervation at the time of major limb amputation in traumatic amputees: early experience of an effective treatment strategy to improve pain. Jbjs Open Access 2020;5(2):e0067.

23. Davidson JH, Khor KE, Jones LE. A cross-sectional study of post-amputation pain in upper and lower limb amputees, experience of a tertiary referral amputee clinic. Disabil Rehabil 2010;32(22):1855–62.

24. Hirsh AT, Dillworth TM, Ehde DM, et al. Sex differences in pain and psychological functioning in persons with limb loss. J Pain 2010;11(1):79–86.

25. Polfer EM, Hoyt BW, Senchak LT, et al. Fluid collections in amputations are not indicative or predictive of infection. Clin Orthop Relat R 2014; 472(10):2978–83.

26. Devers A, Galer BS. Topical lidocaine patch relieves a variety of neuropathic pain conditions: an open-label study. Clin J Pain 2000;16(3):205–8.

27. Nikolajsen L, Hansen CL, Nielsen J, et al. The effect of ketamine on phantom pain: a central neuropathic disorder maintained by peripheral input. Pain 1996;67(1):69–77.

28. Ramachandran VS, Rogers-Ramachandran D. Synaesthesia in phantom limbs induced with mirrors. Proc R Soc Lond Ser B Biol Sci 1996;263(1369):377–86.

29. Poppler LH, Parikh RP, Bichanich MJ, et al. Surgical interventions for the treatment of painful neuroma. Pain 2018;159(2):214–23.

30. Guse DM, Moran SL. Outcomes of the surgical treatment of peripheral neuromas of the hand and forearm. Ann Plast Surg 2013;71(6):654–8.

31. Ives GC, Kung TA, Nghiem BT, et al. Current state of the surgical treatment of terminal neuromas. Neurosurgery 2017;83(3):354–64.

32. Low CK, Chew SH, Song IC, et al. Implantation of a nerve ending into a vein. Clin Orthop Relat R 2000; 379(NA):242–6.

33. Herbert TJ, Filan SL. Vein implantation for treatment of painful cutaneous neuromas A preliminary report. J Hand Surg Br Eur 1998;23(2):220–4.

34. Mobbs RJ, Vonau M, Blum P. Treatment of painful peripheral neuroma by vein implantation. J Clin Neurosci 2003;10(3):338–9.

35. Mass DP, Ciano MC, Tortosa R, et al. Treatment of painful hand neuromas by their transfer into bone. Plast Reconstr Surg 1984;74(2):182–5.

36. Rellan I, Zaidenberg EE, Boretto JG. Bony implantation of neuroma as a possible cause for secondary fractures: a case report. J Hand Surg Eur 2021;46(1): 85–8.

37. Dellon AL, Aszmann OC. In musculus, veritas? Nerve "in muscle" versus targeted muscle reinnervation versus regenerative peripheral nerve interface: historical review. Microsurg 2020;40(4): 516–22.

38. EDDS MV. Prevention of nerve regeneration and neuroma formation by caps of synthetic resin. J Neurosurg 1945;2:507–9.

39. Swanson AB, Boeve NR, Lumsden RM. The prevention and treatment of amputation neuromata by silicone capping. J Hand Surg 1977;2(1):70–8.

40. Galeano M, Manasseri B, Risitano G, et al. A free vein graft cap influences neuroma formation after nerve transection. Microsurg 2009;29(7): 568–72.

41. Fang LD, Jia XH, Wang R, et al. Simulation of the ligament forces affected by prosthetic alignment in a trans-tibial amputee case study. Med Eng Phys 2009;31(7):793–8.

42. Barbera J, Albert-Pamplo R. Centrocentral anastomosis of the proximal nerve stump in the treatment of painful amputation neuromas of major nerves. J Neurosurg 1993;79(3):331–4.

43. Al-Qattan MM. Prevention and treatment of painful neuromas of the superficial radial nerve by the end-to-side nerve repair concept: An experimental study and preliminary clinical experience. Microsurg 2000;20(3):99–104.

44. Aszmann OC, Korak KJ, Rab M, et al. Neuroma prevention by end-to-side neurorraphy: an experimental study in rats1 1No benefits in any form have been received or will be received from a commercial party related directly or indirectly to the subject of this article. J Hand Surg 2003;28(6): 1022–8.

45. Woo SL, Kung TA, Brown DL, et al. Regenerative peripheral nerve interfaces for the treatment of postamputation neuroma pain. Plast Reconstr Surg - Glob Open 2016;4(12):e1038.

46. Hooper RC, Cederna PS, Brown DL, et al. Regenerative peripheral nerve interfaces for the

management of symptomatic hand and digital neuromas. Plast Reconstr Surg - Glob Open 2020;8(6): e2792.

47. Kung TA, Langhals NB, Martin DC, et al. Regenerative peripheral nerve interface viability and signal transduction with an implanted electrode. Plast Reconstr Surg 2014;133(6):1380–94.

48. Geethanjali P. Myoelectric control of prosthetic hands: state-of-the-art review. Med Devices Évid Res. 2016;9:247–55.

49. Langhals NB, Woo SL, Moon JD, et al. Electrically stimulated signals from a long-term regenerative peripheral nerve interface. Annu Int Conf Ieee Eng Med Biol Soc 2014;2014:1989–92. https://doi.org/10.1109/embc.2014.6944004.

50. Nghiem BT, Sando IC, Gillespie RB, et al. Providing a sense of touch to prosthetic hands. Plast Reconstr Surg 2015;135(6):1652–63.

51. Kung TA, Bueno RA, Alkhalefah GK, et al. Innovations in prosthetic interfaces for the upper extremity. Plast Reconstr Surg 2013;132(6):1515–23.

52. Valerio I, Schulz SA, West J, et al. Targeted muscle reinnervation combined with a vascularized pedicled regenerative peripheral nerve interface. Plast Reconstr Surg - Glob Open 2020;8(3):e2689.

53. White TP, Devor ST. Skeletal muscle regeneration and plasticity of grafts. Exerc Sport Sci Revev 1993;21(1):263.

54. Bain JR, Hason Y, Veltri K, et al. Clinical application of sensory protection of denervated muscle: Case report. J Neurosurg 2008;109(5):955–61.

55. Placheta E, Wood MD, Lafontaine C, et al. Enhancement of facial nerve motoneuron regeneration through cross-face nerve grafts by adding end-to-side sensory axons. Plast Reconstr Surg 2015;135(2):460–71.

56. Elsohemy A, Butler R, Bain JR, et al. Sensory protection of rat muscle spindles following peripheral nerve injury and reinnervation. Plast Reconstr Surg 2009;124(6):1860–8.

57. Kubiak CA, Kemp SWP, Cederna PS, et al. Prophylactic regenerative peripheral nerve interfaces to prevent postamputation pain. Plast Reconstr Surg 2019;144(3):421e–30e.

58. Kuiken T, Dumanian G, Lipschutz R, et al. The use of targeted muscle reinnervation for improved myoelectric prosthesis control in a bilateral shoulder disarticulation amputee. Prosthet Orthot Int 2004;(28):245–53.

59. Dumanian GA, Potter BK, Mioton LM, et al. Targeted Muscle Reinnervation Treats Neuroma and Phantom Pain in Major Limb Amputees. Ann Surg 2018;270(2):238–46.

60. Gart MS, Souza JM, Dumanian GA. Targeted muscle reinnervation in the upper extremity amputee: a technical roadmap. J Hand Surg 2015;40(9): 1877–88.

61. Mioton LM, Dumanian GA, Shah N, et al. Targeted muscle reinnervation improves residual limb pain, phantom limb pain, and limb function: a prospective study of 33 major limb Amputees. Clin Orthop Relat Res 2020;478(9):2161–7.

62. Valerio IL, Dumanian GA, Jordan SW, et al. Preemptive treatment of phantom and residual limb pain with targeted muscle reinnervation at the time of major limb amputation. J Am Coll Surg 2019;228(3):217–26.

63. Morgan EN, Potter BK, Souza JM, et al. Targeted muscle reinnervation for transradial amputation. Tech Hand Up Extremity Surg 2016;20(4):166–71.

64. Cheesborough JE, Souza JM, Dumanian GA, et al. Targeted muscle reinnervation in the initial management of traumatic upper extremity amputation injury. Hand 2014;9(2):253–7.

65. Kim PS, Ko JH, O'Shaughnessy KK, et al. The effects of targeted muscle reinnervation on neuromas in a rabbit rectus abdominis flap model. J Hand Surg 2012;37(8):1609–16.

66. Agnew SP, Schultz AE, Dumanian GA, et al. Targeted reinnervation in the transfemoral amputee. Plast Reconstr Surg 2012;129(1):187–94.

67. Bowen JB, Ruter D, Wee C, et al. Targeted muscle reinnervation technique in below-knee amputation. Plast Reconstr Surg 2019;143(1):309–12.

68. Dumanian GA, Ko JH, O'Shaughnessy KD, et al. Targeted reinnervation for transhumeral amputees: current surgical technique and update on results. Plast Reconstr Surg 2009;124(3):863–9.

Pediatrics

Brachial Plexus Birth Injuries

James S. Lin, MD[a], Julie Balch Samora, MD, PhD[a,b,*]

KEYWORDS

- Brachial plexus birth injury • Pediatrics • Nerve injury • Nerve surgery
- Obstetric brachial plexus palsy

KEY POINTS

- Brachial plexus birth injuries remain fairly common in the United States, occurring in approximately 0.9 per 1000 live births.
- Spontaneous recovery can be expected in the majority of cases. Serial clinical examination remains the gold standard for evaluation and initial management.
- Indications for early surgical intervention by 3 months of age include cases of total plexopathy, Horner syndrome, and root avulsion. Otherwise, it is generally reasonable to continue nonsurgical management until about 6 months of age.
- Many surgical techniques have been described. Neurolysis alone is no longer recommended, and direct nerve repair is rarely possible due to tension on the repair construct. The most common surgical finding is a neuroma in continuity, and neuroma resection and nerve grafting are often performed. Nerve transfers are gaining in popularity, with promising results, including when performed later in life (1–2 years of age). Osseous procedures such as derotational humeral osteotomy can also be performed in cases of significant glenohumeral dysplasia.

INTRODUCTION/RISK FACTORS

Brachial plexus birth injuries (BPBIs) are typically traction type injuries to the newborn that occur during the delivery process. Although the incidence of these injuries has overall decreased from 1.5 to around 0.9 per 1000 live births in the United States over the past 2 decades, these injuries remain common, with incidence holding fairly steady from 2008 to 2014.[1–4] Shoulder dystocia is the strongest identified risk factor, imparting a 100-fold greater risk.[1,5] The newborn's shoulder is caught behind the mother's pubic bone, and traction performed on the child during delivery results in injury to the brachial plexus. Other risk factors associated with BPBI include macrosomia (birthweight > 4.5 kg), heavy for gestational age infants, birth hypoxia,

gestational diabetes, and forceps or vacuum-assisted delivery.[1,5,6] Breech presentation has also been described as a risk factor in the past, but there have been more recent data that challenge this association.[1,2,7–9]

Protective factors include multiple gestation and cesarean section delivery.[1,5] Of note, rates of cesarean section delivery has consistently increased over the last 2 decades, which may make the risk factors of shoulder dystocia and instrument-assisted delivery less relevant in the future.[1,2,10] However, more than 50% of cases have no identified risk factors.[1,5] Therefore, it has been proposed that alternative risk factors may account for these largely consistent rates of BPBI, especially in the setting of increasing cesarean delivery rates.[2,4] For instance, relative hypotonia—due to fetal distress—is a more

---

[a] Department of Orthopaedics, The Ohio State University Wexner Medical Center, 700 Children's Drive, T2E-A2700, Columbus, OH 43205, USA; [b] Department of Orthopedic Surgery, Nationwide Children's Hopsital, Columbus, OH, USA
* Corresponding author.
E-mail address: julie.samora@nationwidechildrens.org

Orthop Clin N Am 53 (2022) 167–177
https://doi.org/10.1016/j.ocl.2021.11.003
0030-5898/22/© 2021 Elsevier Inc. All rights reserved.

recently recognized risk factor as it leads to less protection of the brachial plexus during delivery, making it more susceptible to stretch injury.[2,8] In addition, oxytocin use and uterine tachysystole (defined as greater than 5 contractions in a 10 minute period) have been recently identified factors that contribute to BPBI.[7,11]

CLASSIFICATION BY DEGREE OF NERVE INJURY

Understanding the types of nerve injury is helpful to determine the management and prognosis for BPBI. According to the Seddon classification system, neuropraxia is the mildest form of injury, whereby the nerve roots sustain a stretch or compression injury that results in focal demyelination without the disruption of axon continuity. Neuropraxic injuries have the best prognosis, and complete recovery can be expected generally within the first 2 months of life.[7,12] Axonotmesis occurs when the axons are severed but the epineurium remains intact.[13] These injuries have been further classified into 3 types by Sunderland, as they have widely varying degrees of severity and recovery potential depending on the involvement of the surrounding nerve structures such as the endoneurium and perineurium.[14] Neurotmesis injuries are the most severe of the Seddon classification, as they represent a physiologic disruption of the entire nerve with spontaneous recovery being very unlikely.[13] Finally, avulsions of the brachial plexus root from the spinal cord itself are preganglionic lesions, which are devastating injuries with poor potential for recovery without surgical intervention.[7,15]

CLASSIFICATION BY CLINICAL PRESENTATION

The brachial plexus consists of the ventral nerve roots of C5 through T1, which provide all sensory and motor functions for the upper extremity.[16] Variation has been reported in the literature, with approximately 22% of cases having prefixed cords in which C4 also provided contribution. In this study, there was also one case in which C4-T2 comprised the plexus and another case for which the plexus was comprised of C5-C8.[17] The C5 and C6 nerve roots comprise the upper trunk and are largely involved in shoulder and elbow flexion and supination. C7 becomes the middle trunk which primarily controls elbow extension. C8 and T1 form the lower trunk, which is involved in hand function.[8,18] These trunks each divide into anterior and posterior divisions that consolidate to form three cords (lateral, posterior, and medial), which further divide into branches.

Around 60% of BPBI cases are of the upper plexus (C5 and C6), known as Erb palsy.[7] These cases exhibit the classic "waiter's tip" position with the shoulder internally rotated, elbow extended, and wrist flexed and pronated due to deficits in the muscles innervated by the C5 and C6 nerve roots: deltoid, supraspinatus, infraspinatus, teres minor, elbow flexors, and wrist extensors.[19] These types of injuries are clinically the mildest and have the best prognosis, with spontaneous recovery occurring in about 90% of cases.[20] 20% to 30% of cases are considered extended Erb palsy, which involves C5, C6, and C7. In these cases, the shoulder internal rotators, triceps, and finger extensors are deficient as well, and the elbow may rest in a slightly flexed posture.[21] With extended Erb palsy, children may have midline function deficits, making self-care and perineal hygiene more challenging.[22]

Lower root injury is characterized by Klumpke palsy, which involves the C8 and T1 nerve roots. These injuries are rare, accounting for less than 1% of cases.[7] Children with these injuries have deficits in their hand flexors and intrinsics.[16] Klumpke palsy may also present following a case of total plexus palsy that had recovery of the upper trunk but incomplete recovery of the C8 and T1 nerve roots. Total plexus palsies, which involve C5 – T1, account for 15% to 20% of cases and present as no upper extremity function. These cases have the worst prognosis.[7,16] Horner syndrome is frequently associated with lower root avulsions (C8 and T1) and therefore typically present in patients with Klumpke palsy and total plexopathy.[23] However, cases of Horner syndrome have also been described in patients with extended Erb palsy.[24] This syndrome of ipsilateral ptosis, miosis, and anhidrosis indicates injury to the sympathetic nerves of the face, and its presence is associated with worse prognosis for recovery of the plexopathy.[24,25]

The Narakas classification[26] system excludes many mild cases that resolve within days, and it characterizes injuries by levels of severity and potential for spontaneous recovery. For instance, Narakas group I injuries are the most mild, and they include infants that present with Erb palsy. In this series, all patients in group I recovered good shoulder function.[26] Narakas group II injuries include cases of extended Erb palsy, as these are more severe injuries. In Narakas group III patients, nearly the entire upper extremity is affected. Narakas group IV patients have total plexopathy with paralysis of the C5 – T1 roots with associated Horner syndrome. No patients in group IV had spontaneous recovery of function.[26]

PATIENT EVALUATION OVERVIEW

BPBI is often immediately apparent at the time of birth, as the parent or provider notices no arm movement in the newborn. Physical examination remains the gold standard for diagnosis, and serial examinations provide valuable information on prognosis.[27] Electrodiagnostic testing has not been shown to have value in providing prognostic information, as compensatory movements and multiple innervations of muscles make interpretation of these studies difficult.[28] Advanced imaging with computed tomography (CT) myelography and magnetic resonance imaging (MRI) are commonly used modalities in adult brachial plexus injuries. These studies can differentiate between avulsion and rupture as well as reveal pseudomeningocele. The principal limitation in these studies is that they are difficult to obtain in BPBI, as these patients require general anesthesia, and placement of intrathecal contrast dye for infants may be challenging.[27] However, a three-dimensional proton density MRI has been recently described, which is able to evaluate spinal nerve roots in infants held in a vacuum-suction controlled positioner without the need for sedation, radiation, or contrast.[29]

ASSOCIATED FRACTURES

Associated injuries are important to rule out in cases of BPBI. If osseous injury is suspected, radiographs are indicated because fractures can mimic palsy or occur concomitantly with BPBI.[7,30] For instance, clavicular fractures are more prevalent in the setting of BPBIs at an incidence of around 8% to 9% compared with an incidence of 0.3% of all births.[31,32] However, a recent population study found that the presence of clavicular fractures is not independently correlated with BPBI in infants with shoulder dystocia.[32] Furthermore, there is no consensus on the prognostic value of a concomitant clavicular fracture in the setting of BPBI. One retrospective study has suggested that the presence of clavicular fracture may be protective of neurologic recovery in BPBI.[33] However, other studies report that clavicle fractures have not been shown to be predictive of BPBI severity or need for microsurgical intervention.[31,34]

Humerus fractures at birth may mimic BPBI, as the newborn will avoid the movement of the entire extremity due to pain. It has been suggested that humeral fractures are rare in the setting of an ipsilateral BPBI, as humeral shaft fractures are more likely to result in an isolated radial nerve palsy.[35–37] However, a recent study has found that the incidence of humerus fractures in the setting of BPBI may be as high as 7%.[31]

ASSESSMENT SCALES

There are several clinical scoring systems that have been shown to reliably assess upper extremity function in BPBI.[38] The Hospital for Sick Children Active Movement Scale (AMS) scores 15 different active upper extremity movements against gravity and also with gravity eliminated (Table 1).[39] Each movement receives a score from 0 to 7, and scores of less than 4.5 at 3 months of age specifically for elbow extension, wrist extension, and finger, thumb, and wrist flexion were found to be independent predictors for patients requiring microsurgical intervention.[40]

The Toronto Test Score evaluates 5 movements—elbow flexion, and elbow, wrist, thumb, and finger extension against gravity—on a scale of 0 to 2, whereby 0 = no movement and 2 = full range of movement.[41] All 5-movement scores are combined into an aggregate score from 0 to 10. A score > 3.5 at 3 months of age suggests good recovery without surgical intervention.[41]

The Mallet classification scores 5 different shoulder movements: global abduction, global external rotation, hand behind neck, hand as high as possible up the spine, and hand to mouth.[42] The classification grades each movement from Grade I to Grade V, whereby I = no function and V = normal function. There have been concerns that the original Mallet scale is biased toward external rotation, and therefore Abzug and colleagues[43] proposed the addition of a sixth category of hand to navel movement. This additional component provides another assessment of internal rotation and insight on midline function which is critical for daily function and hygiene, which has garnered broad support (Fig. 1).[43,44] Although all 3 scoring systems individually have been validated to have good reliability,[38] the correlation between the modified Mallet classification and either the AMS or Toronto scores is poor.[44] Therefore, these scoring systems should not be used interchangeably to guide clinical decision-making for children with BPBI.

Table 1 Active movement scale	
Observation	**Score**
Gravity eliminated	
No contraction	0
Contraction, no motion	1
$\leq$ 50% total passive range of motion	2
> 50% total passive range of motion	3
Full range of motion	4
Against Gravity	
$\leq$ 50% total passive range of motion	5
> 50% total passive range of motion	6
Full range of motion	7

NONSURGICAL MANAGEMENT

Given the potential for spontaneous recovery in most of cases, nonsurgical treatment is the initial management strategy. Therapy with passive range of motion of the entire extremity is initiated to prevent contractures. Stabilization of the scapulothoracic joint is performed to facilitate glenohumeral motion in these patients, as children with BPBI have disproportionately greater motion of the scapulothoracic joint compared with the glenohumeral joint.[8] The inverse is exhibited in unaffected shoulders, with a 2:1 ratio of glenohumeral to scapulothoracic movement.[45,46]

TIMING OF SURGICAL MANAGEMENT

The primary indication for surgical intervention is a lack of spontaneous recovery of function on serial physical examinations. Timing remains controversial. Knowledge of the true natural history of BPBI is limited, as an investigation would require withholding treatment that has been demonstrated to improve outcomes.[35,47] Furthermore, well-powered prospective randomized studies are difficult to perform given the heterogeneity of lesions and highly variable preferences in treatment approaches.[48,49]

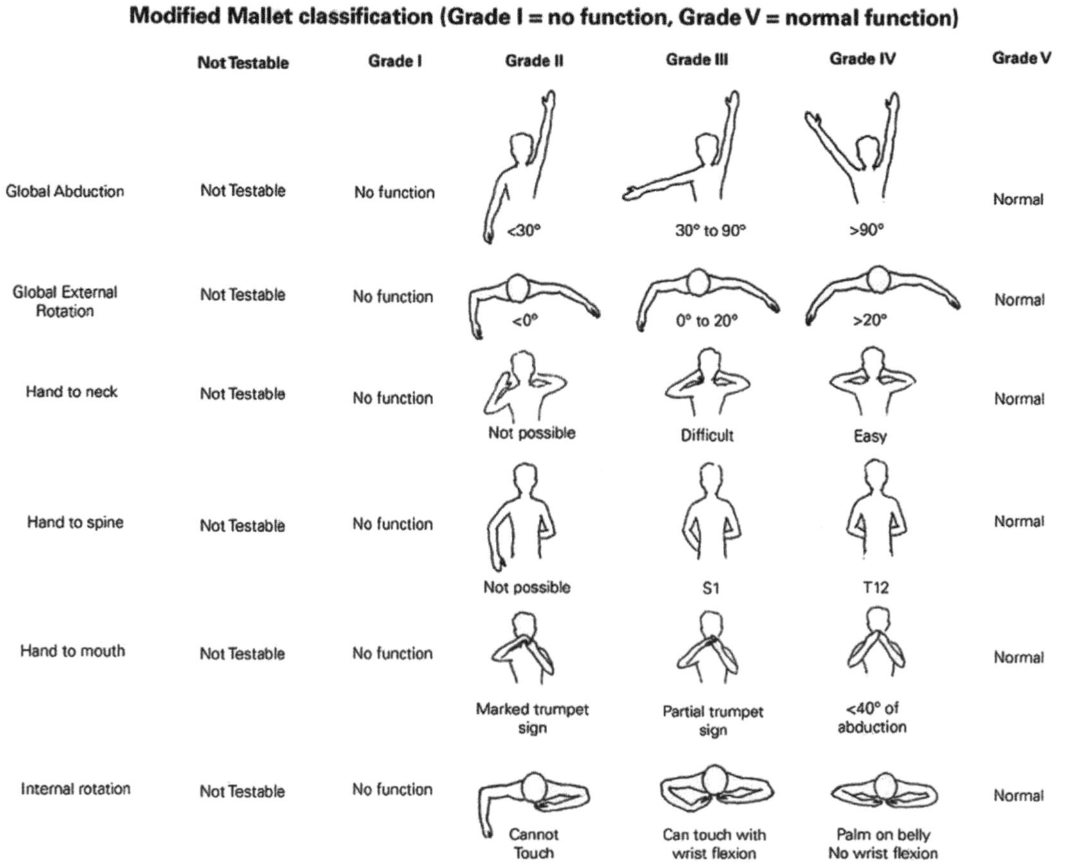

Fig. 1. Modified Mallet Classification to assess upper extremity function whereby Grade I = no function and grade V = normal function. (*Courtesy of* Shriners Hospital for Children, Philadelphia, PA)

Nevertheless, there has been fair evidence (level II or III studies with consistent findings[50]) to support early operative intervention (by 3 months of age) for cases of total plexopathy, Horner syndrome, and root avulsion injuries.[27]

For patients who do not fit into those categories, there is less consensus. Surgical exploration and reconstruction are recommended by the classic teaching by Gilbert and colleagues[51] for patients without active biceps contraction or elbow flexion at 3 months of age because these patients were unlikely to regain normal shoulder function, which has been supported by other series.[52] In contrast, Smith and colleagues found that two-thirds (8/12) of patients in their series with C5-C6 injuries without biceps function at 3 months still developed good shoulder function without surgical intervention.[53] To further complicate things, surgical intervention has also been found to improve function in certain patients who *did* have elbow flexion at 3 months.[54,55] Therefore, the presence or absence of elbow flexion at 3 months alone is likely insufficient to make surgical decisions.

One treatment algorithm based on the Hospital for Sick Children protocol uses serial examinations and specific indications at different timepoints (Fig. 2).[54] Surgery is recommended for patients at 3 months of age with Toronto Test Scores < 3.5 and those with T1 avulsion and/or Horner syndrome. A "cookie test" is administered at 9 months of age, a test that evaluates the midline function of the patient by their ability to bring a cookie to their mouth without significant compensatory movement of the neck.[39] Operative intervention is recommended if the patient is unable to perform the test. Surgery may also be recommended at 6 months of age if there is no significant progress since the 3-month assessment and they are unlikely to pass the cookie test at 9 months.[54]

A multicenter prospective study recently published by the treatment and outcomes of brachial plexus injury (TOBI) Study Group found no difference in outcomes between microsurgical intervention performed before and after 6 months of age when controlled for injury severity.[56] These authors did assert that the timepoint at which it becomes too late to attempt motor reinnervation remains unknown. They also found overall improvements in function when nerve reconstruction was performed in children over the age of 9 months.[57] The TOBI group concludes that expected functional recovery cannot be the sole factor in deciding whether or not to proceed with surgery. For instance, surgical intervention may be technically

easier to perform for younger infants as there is less neuroma formation and shorter distances that need to be covered by nerve grafts.[56]

However, a cost-effectiveness analysis demonstrated that performing surgery at 3 months incurs over twice as much overall costs than if surgery were performed at 6 months of age. This cost differential stems from the greater number of patients who would undergo surgical intervention if offered at an earlier age. These authors concluded that surgery performed at 3 months of age is unlikely to produce enough improvement in quality of life compared with surgery at 6 months of age to justify the greater costs.[58] Taken together, it may be reasonable to continue nonsurgical management until six months of age for children with brachial plexus birth injuries without Horner syndrome, avulsion injuries, plexopathy, as waiting until this timepoint does not seem to adversely affect outcomes.[27]

SURGICAL TECHNIQUES

The goal of nerve surgery is to facilitate the reinnervation of the affected muscles of the upper extremity. The spectrum of microsurgical techniques includes neurolysis, neuroma excision, interpositional nerve grafting and conduits, and nerve transfers.[59] Direct nerve repair is rarely an option because of the inability to prevent undue tension at the repair site without grafting.[35] Nevertheless, direct repair following neuroma resection early in life has been reported to have favorable outcomes.[60]

Neurolysis is a controversial strategy. It involves the exploration of the plexus and excision of scar tissue. It has been well established that this technique does not play a role in patients with total plexopathy or root avulsion injures.[61] The most common finding in cases of BPBI is a neuroma in continuity of the upper trunk at the confluence of the C5-C6 roots.[59] Historically, neurolysis was described to be an option for patients with neuromas in continuity with sufficient conduction through the neuroma (defined as <50% amplitude drop of muscle action potential).[62] Initially, there were favorable outcomes found in neurolysis of neuromas in continuity at 12-months postoperatively for patients with Erb palsy.[61] However, these functional improvements were not sustained over time, and the same authors now contend there is no role for neurolysis alone, a notion that has been supported by other groups.[21,63]

Neuroma resection and nerve grafting has been advocated in lieu of neurolysis due to superior outcomes.[63,64] Specifically, autologous sural

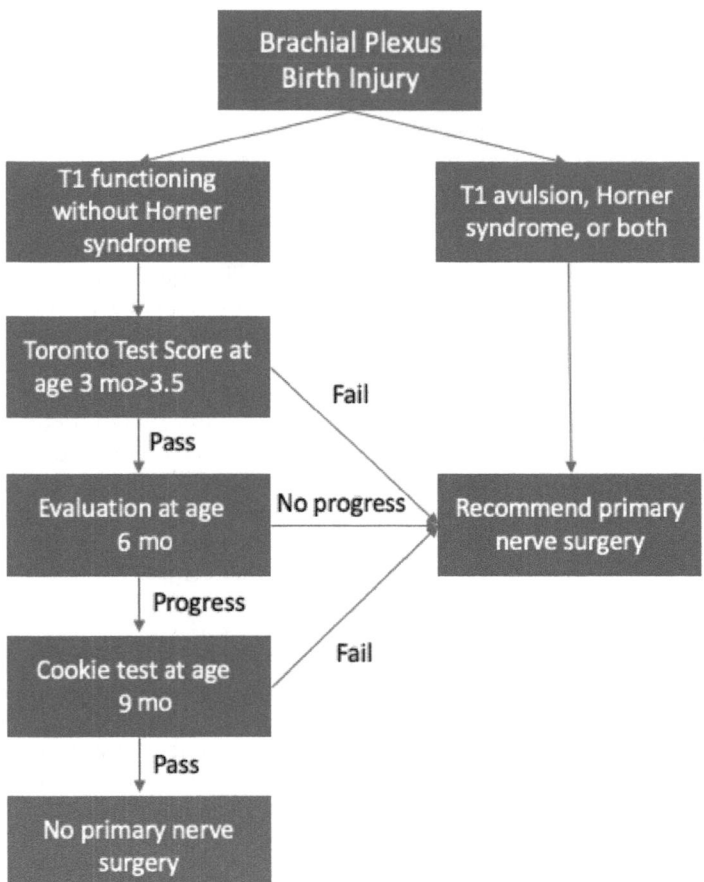

Fig. 2. Hospital for Sick Children treatment algorithm of indications for primary nerve surgery in brachial plexus birth injury (revised Hospital for Sick Children algorithm). (*Adapted from* Bade SA, Lin JC, Curtis CG, et al. Extending the indications for primary nerve surgery in obstetric brachial plexus palsy. Biomed Res Int 2014;2014:627067.)

nerve grafts are most commonly used.[27,35,65] Processed allografts and collagen nerve conduits have been proposed for their advantages of decreased operative time and donor site morbidity, but their efficacy has yet to be proven in cases of BPBI.[35] An animal model has demonstrated that autograft still had superior outcomes in motor recovery than allograft or conduit.[66]

Nerve transfers have been increasing in use. This technique has been well established for traumatic brachial plexus injuries in adults, as it affords advantages over traditional nerve grafting such as proximity of the donor's nerve to the denervated muscle endplates as well as faster operative and recovery times.[67,68] Its role in BPBI is gaining popularity. Ladak and colleagues published a series of patients aged 10 to 18 months with isolated upper trunk injuries who underwent 3 nerve transfers.[68] Specifically, a branch of the spinal accessory nerve was transferred to the suprascapular nerve; a motor branch of the radial nerve to the axillary nerve; and a motor branch of the ulnar nerve to the

musculocutaneous nerve (known as the Oberlin transfer[69]) to provide shoulder abduction and external rotation, shoulder abduction, and elbow flexion, respectively. These authors found significant improvements in function sustained at 2-years postoperatively, comparable to those achieved with nerve grafting.[68] Similarly, the prospective series by Daly and colleagues and the TOBI Study Group found similar outcomes for patients who underwent a variety of nerve transfers and for those who underwent nerve grafting after 9 months of age.[57] These authors asserted that a recommendation supporting one technique over the other cannot be made. However, the same study group also compared spinal accessory to suprascapular nerve transfer versus nerve grafting to the suprascapular nerve, finding that the transfer group was more likely to achieve functional shoulder external rotation (AMS score > 5) and have fewer secondary shoulder procedures.[70]

One should be cognizant that nerve transfer is not benign with donor site morbidity likely underreported.[71] In addition, this technique does not provide sensory reinnervation, and the long-term consequences to the extremity are unknown.[72] Nevertheless, there are circumstances in which nerve transfers are the only option. In preganglionic injuries such as root avulsions, nerve transfers are required, as nerve grafting is not possible due to the lack of proximal roots.[73] Indications for distal nerve transfers include late presentation (1–2 years of age), whereby there is insufficient time for axonal growth to support nerve grafting.[72] Al-Qattan published the first report of using the Oberlin transfer for BPBI in 2 infants who presented at 16 and 18 months with Erb palsy, and both patients successfully achieved normal elbow function by 5-months postoperatively.[74] Larger series have also demonstrated the success of nerve transfer in BPBI up to 26 months of age, although younger patients demonstrated greater recovery of supination.[75–77] Additional indications for nerve transfer include failed nerve grafting, as donor roots have already been used, and dissociative recovery, whereby upper trunk function recovers for the shoulder but not for elbow flexion.[76,78]

SECONDARY PROCEDURES

Secondary procedures may be required to address musculoskeletal pathology associated with BPBI. Commonly, glenohumeral dysplasia can occur due to muscle imbalance resulting in strong internal rotation and weak external rotation forces on the shoulder. This imparts a posteriorly directed force on the glenohumeral joint, leading to progressive glenoid retroversion and posterior subluxation of the humeral head.[8] In fact, there is a 7% incidence of posterior shoulder dislocation in children with BPBI under 1 year of age.[79] Therefore, it is critical to screen all patients with BPBI for shoulder dislocation, with lack passive external rotation of the shoulder indicating underlying joint deformity. Specifically, patients with less than 60° of passive external rotation in adduction should undergo further evaluation with ultrasound or MRI to evaluate for shoulder dislocation.

A number of treatment and prevention strategies have been proposed. Early therapy with passive range of motion exercises can be performed to prevent or improve contractures.[8] There is also a role for orthoses, as extension wrist splints and supinator traps to the forearm can help the extremity rest in more neutral positions.[80] The use of botulinum toxin to temporarily weaken the strong internal rotators of the shoulder has also been described to help maintain a reduction in infants with early posterior shoulder subluxation or dislocation due to BPBI.[80,81] The addition of posterior capsulorrhaphy has also been found to improve shoulder function.[82,83] Subscapularis release can be considered for those who have a persistent internal rotation contracture.[84–86] While older patients may ultimately require a derotational humeral osteotomy,[8] there are data that suggest open reduction and subscapularis lengthening can facilitate the remodeling of glenohumeral dysplasia for patients with BPBI up to 5 years of age.[86]

Simultaneous tendon transfers at the time of an anterior release and open reduction can also be used. Specifically, extra-articular transfers of the latissimus dorsi and teres major to the insertion of the supraspinatus and infraspinatus have been shown to aid forward flexion, abduction, and external rotation as well as slow progression of glenohumeral deformity.[87] Waters and Bae[88] demonstrated that open reduction in combination with tendon transfers and anterior lengthening improved shoulder function and glenohumeral remodeling for 19 of 23 (83%) patients (aged 8–50 months) at a mean follow-up of 31 months. Of these patients, 20 were available for intermediate-term follow-up, and a recently published study found that the improvements were sustained. However, the greatest improvements in radiographic measurements occurred within the first year postoperatively, and there were no significant changes in shoulder function or radiographic outcomes beyond the first year.[89] Of note, these authors do contend that inadequate power is likely precluded them from detecting statistical significance.

Osseous procedures such as humeral derotational osteotomy are typically indicated for a child with persistent external rotation deficits despite prior soft tissue procedures and/or those with advanced progressive glenohumeral dysplasia, whereby tendon transfer and contracture release alone are inadequate to correct the deficits in external rotation.[8,90] Forty-three patients underwent derotational humeral osteotomy at a mean age of 7.6 years, achieving overall improvements in shoulder function.[90] Various techniques have been described, including a percutaneous osteotomy with osteosynthesis by an external fixation system.[91]

An emerging technique is glenoid anteversion osteotomy, which can be performed concomitantly with soft tissue balancing in lieu of external rotation osteotomy of the humerus.[92,93] Early results have been positive, with improvements in function and maintenance of joint reduction. Furthermore, there are secondary procedures that address deformity of the elbow and forearm. For instance, radial and ulnar osteotomies along with biceps tendon transfer can be used to improve forearm supination and elbow flexion contractures—which may be observed in cases of C7 – T1 weakness.[8,94]

SUMMARY

Although spontaneous recovery can be expected in most cases of BPBIs, some patients require surgical intervention to improve their upper extremity function. Specific indications exist for early nerve surgery by 3 months of age. Otherwise, patients have generally had favorable outcomes with various surgical techniques including nerve grafting, nerve and tendon transfers, and osteotomies at 6 months of age or later. High-quality comparative studies have been limited due to the wide spectrum of injury types, treatment techniques, and surgeon preferences. However, emerging long-term data from multicenter studies have shown promise in treatment options for these patients.

CLINICS CARE POINTS

- Physical examination is the gold standard for diagnosis of brachial plexus birth injuries, and serial examinations provide valuable information on prognosis

- Given the potential for spontaneous recovery in the majority of cases, nonsurgical treatment is often the initial management strategy

- The primary indication for surgical intervention is a lack of spontaneous recovery of function on serial physical examinations

- Optimal timing of surgery remains controversial, but level II and III studies support early operative intervention (by 3 months of age) for cases of total plexopathy, Horner syndrome, and root avulsion injuries

- For children with brachial plexus birth injuries who do not fall into these severe categories, it may be reasonable to continue nonsurgical management until 6 months of age, as waiting until this timepoint does not seem to adversely affect outcomes

- Common surgical interventions include neuroma resection and nerve grafting as well as nerve transfers.

DISCLOSURE

The authors have no relevant disclosures.

REFERENCES

1. Foad SL, Mehlman CT, Ying J. The epidemiology of neonatal brachial plexus palsy in the United States. J Bone Joint Surg Am 2008;90(6):1258–64.
2. Abzug JM, Mehlman CT, Ying J. Assessment of current epidemiology and risk factors surrounding brachial plexus birth palsy. J Hand Surg Am 2019; 44(6):515.e1–10.
3. Gupta R, Cabacungan ET. Neonatal birth trauma: analysis of yearly trends, risk factors, and outcomes. J Pediatr 2021. https://doi.org/10.1016/j.jpeds.2021.06.080.
4. Walsh JM, Kandamany N, Ni Shuibhne N, et al. Neonatal brachial plexus injury: comparison of incidence and antecedents between 2 decades. Am J Obstet Gynecol 2011;204(4):324.e1–6.
5. DeFrancesco CJ, Shah DK, Rogers BH, et al. The epidemiology of brachial plexus birth palsy in the United States: declining incidence and evolving risk factors. J Pediatr Orthop 2019;39(2):e134–40.
6. Al-Qattan MM, El-Sayed AA, Al-Zahrani AY, et al. Obstetric brachial plexus palsy in newborn babies of diabetic and non-diabetic mothers. J Hand Surg Eur 2010;35(5):362–5.
7. Abzug JM, Kozin SH. Evaluation and management of brachial plexus birth palsy. Orthop Clin North Am 2014;45(2):225–32.
8. Waters PM. Obstetric Brachial Plexus Injuries: Evaluation and Management. J Am Acad Orthop Surg 1997;5(4):205–14.
9. Sibiński M, Synder M. Obstetric brachial plexus palsy–risk factors and predictors. Ortop Traumatol Rehabil 2007;9(6):569–76.
10. Sebastião YV, Womack L, Vamos CA, et al. Hospital variation in cesarean delivery rates: contribution of individual and hospital factors in Florida. Am J Obstet Gynecol 2016;214(1):123.e1–18.
11. Louden E, Marcotte M, Mehlman C, et al. Risk Factors for Brachial Plexus Birth Injury. Children (Basel) 2018;5(4). https://doi.org/10.3390/children5040046.
12. Seddon HJ. A Classification of Nerve Injuries. Br Med J 1942;2(4260):237–9.
13. Lee SK, Wolfe SW. Peripheral nerve injury and repair. J Am Acad Orthop Surg 2000;8(4):243–52.
14. Sunderland S. Nerve injuries and their repair. Edinburgh, Churchill Livingstone: A Critical Reappraisal; 1991.
15. Kawai H, Kawabata H, Masada K, et al. Nerve repairs for traumatic brachial plexus palsy with root avulsion. Clin Orthop Relat Res 1988;(237):75–86.
16. Yang LJ-S, McGillicuddy JE, Chimbira W. Clinical presentation and considerations of neonatal brachial

plexus palsy. Practical management of pediatric and adult brachial plexus palsies e-book. 2011:35.

17. Lee HY, Chung IH, Sir WS, et al. Variations of the ventral rami of the brachial plexus. J Korean Med Sci 1992;7(1):19–24.

18. Felten D, O'Banion M, Maida M. Peripheral nervous system. Netter's Atlas of neuroscience. 3rd edition. Amsterdam (The Netherlands): Elsevier; 2016. p. 153–231.

19. Geutjens G, Gilbert A, Helsen K. Obstetric brachial plexus palsy associated with breech delivery. A different pattern of injury. J Bone Joint Surg Br 1996;78(2):303–6.

20. Slooff AC. Obstetric brachial plexus lesions and their neurosurgical treatment. Clin Neurol Neurosurg 1993;95(Suppl):S73–7.

21. Gilbert A, Whitaker I. Obstetrical brachial plexus lesions. J Hand Surg Br 1991;16(5):489–91.

22. Adidharma W, Lewis SP, Liu Y, et al. Shoulder release and tendon transfer following neonatal brachial plexus palsy: gains, losses, and midline function. Plast Reconstr Surg 2020;146(2): 321–31.

23. Al-Qattan MM, Clarke HM, Curtis CG. The prognostic value of concurrent Horner's syndrome in total obstetric brachial plexus injury. J Hand Surg Br 2000;25(2):166–7.

24. El-Sayed AA. The prognostic value of concurrent Horner syndrome in extended Erb obstetric brachial plexus palsy. J Child Neurol 2014;29(10):1356–9.

25. Gosk J, Koszewicz M, Urban M, et al. Assessment of the prognostic value of horner syndrome in perinatal brachial plexus palsy. Neuropediatrics 2011; 42(1):4–6.

26. Narakas A. Obstetrical brachial plexus injury. Edinburgh, Churchill Livingstone: The paralyzed hand; 1987.

27. Pulos N, Shaughnessy WJ, Spinner RJ, et al. Brachial plexus birth injuries: a critical analysis review. JBJS Rev 2021;9(6). https://doi.org/10.2106/JBJS.RVW.20.00004.

28. Heise CO, Siqueira MG, Martins RS, et al. Clinical-electromyography correlation in infants with obstetric brachial plexopathy. J Hand Surg Am 2007; 32(7):999–1004.

29. Bauer AS, Shen PY, Nidecker AE, et al. Neonatal magnetic resonance imaging without sedation correlates with injury severity in brachial plexus birth palsy. J Hand Surg Am 2017;42(5):335–43.

30. Verhees RA, Besselaar AT, van Aken MH, et al. [A neonatal supracondylar humeral fracture resembling a plexus injury]. Ned Tijdschr Geneeskd 2016;160:A9427.

31. Leshikar HB, Bauer AS, Lightdale-Miric N, et al, TOBI Study Group. Clavicle fracture is not predictive of the need for microsurgery in brachial plexus birth palsy. J Pediatr Orthop 2018;38(2):128–32.

32. Gandhi RA, DeFrancesco CJ, Shah AS. The association of clavicle fracture with brachial plexus birth palsy. J Hand Surg Am 2019;44(6):467–72.

33. Wall LB, Mills JK, Leveno K, et al. Incidence and prognosis of neonatal brachial plexus palsy with and without clavicle fractures. Obstet Gynecol 2014;123(6):1288–93.

34. al-Qattan MM, Clarke HM, Curtis CG. The prognostic value of concurrent clavicular fractures in newborns with obstetric brachial plexus palsy. J Hand Surg Br 1994;19(6):729–30.

35. Cornwall R, Waters P. Pediatric brachial plexus palsy. Green's operative hand surgery. Philadelphia (PA): Elsevier; 2017. p. 1391–424.

36. Alsubhi FS, Althunyan AM, Curtis CG, et al. Radial nerve palsy in the newborn: a case series. CMAJ 2011;183(12):1367–70.

37. Mahapatra SK, Jangira V, Kalra M. Neonatal radial nerve palsy associated with humerus fracture: is the fracture to be blamed? Orthop Surg 2014;6(2): 162–4.

38. Bae DS, Waters PM, Zurakowski D. Reliability of three classification systems measuring active motion in brachial plexus birth palsy. J Bone Joint Surg Am 2003;85(9):1733–8.

39. Clarke HM, Curtis CG. An approach to obstetrical brachial plexus injuries. Hand Clin 1995;11(4): 563–80 [discussion: 580-1].

40. Shah AS, Kalish LA, Bae DS, et al. Early predictors of microsurgical reconstruction in brachial plexus birth palsy. Iowa Orthop J 2019;39(1):37–43.

41. Michelow BJ, Clarke HM, Curtis CG, et al. The natural history of obstetrical brachial plexus palsy. Plast Reconstr Surg 1994;93(4):675–80 [discussion: 681].

42. Mallet J. [Obstetrical paralysis of the brachial plexus. II. Therapeutics. Treatment of sequelae. Priority for the treatment of the shoulder. Method for the expression of results]. Rev Chir Orthop Reparatrice Appar Mot 1972;58(Suppl 1):166–8.

43. Abzug JM, Chafetz RS, Gaughan JP, et al. Shoulder function after medial approach and derotational humeral osteotomy in patients with brachial plexus birth palsy. J Pediatr Orthop 2010;30(5):469–74.

44. Greenhill DA, Lukavsky R, Tomlinson-Hansen S, et al. Relationships between 3 classification systems in brachial plexus birth palsy. J Pediatr Orthop 2017;37(6):374–80.

45. Duff SV, Dayanidhi S, Kozin SH. Asymmetrical shoulder kinematics in children with brachial plexus birth palsy. Clin Biomech (Bristol, Avon) 2007;22(6): 630–8.

46. Kumar VP. Biomechanics of the shoulder. Ann Acad Med Singap 2002;31(5):590–2.

47. Pondaag W, Malessy MJ. The evidence for nerve repair in obstetric brachial plexus palsy revisited. Biomed Res Int 2014;2014:434619.

48. Belzberg AJ, Dorsi MJ, Storm PB, et al. Surgical repair of brachial plexus injury: a multinational survey of experienced peripheral nerve surgeons. J Neurosurg 2004;101(3):365–76.

49. Bodensteiner JB, Rich KM, Landau WM. Early infantile surgery for birth-related brachial plexus injuries: justification requires a prospective controlled study. J Child Neurol 1994;9(2):109–10.

50. Wright JG. Revised grades of recommendation for summaries or reviews of orthopaedic surgical studies. J Bone Joint Surg Am 2006;88(5):1161–2.

51. Gilbert A, Brockman R, Carlioz H. Surgical treatment of brachial plexus birth palsy. Clin Orthop Relat Res 1991;(264):39–47.

52. Waters PM. Comparison of the natural history, the outcome of microsurgical repair, and the outcome of operative reconstruction in brachial plexus birth palsy. J Bone Joint Surg Am 1999;81(5):649–59.

53. Smith NC, Rowan P, Benson LJ, et al. Neonatal brachial plexus palsy. Outcome of absent biceps function at three months of age. J Bone Joint Surg Am 2004;86(10):2163–70.

54. Bade SA, Lin JC, Curtis CG, et al. Extending the indications for primary nerve surgery in obstetrical brachial plexus palsy. Biomed Res Int 2014;2014: 627067.

55. Fisher DM, Borschel GH, Curtis CG, et al. Evaluation of elbow flexion as a predictor of outcome in obstetrical brachial plexus palsy. Plast Reconstr Surg 2007;120(6):1585–90.

56. Bauer AS, Kalish LA, Adamczyk MJ, et al. Microsurgery for Brachial Plexus Injury Before Versus After 6 Months of Age: Results of the Multicenter Treatment and Outcomes of Brachial Plexus Injury (TOBI) Study. J Bone Joint Surg Am 2020;102(3): 194–204.

57. Daly MC, Bauer AS, Lynch H, et al, Group TaOoBP-BITS. Outcomes of Late Microsurgical Nerve Reconstruction for Brachial Plexus Birth Injury. J Hand Surg Am 2020;45(6):555.e1–9.

58. Brauer CA, Waters PM. An economic analysis of the timing of microsurgical reconstruction in brachial plexus birth palsy. J Bone Joint Surg Am 2007; 89(5):970–8.

59. Hale HB, Bae DS, Waters PM. Current concepts in the management of brachial plexus birth palsy. J Hand Surg Am 2010;35(2):322–31.

60. Kirjavainen M, Remes V, Peltonen J, et al. Long-term results of surgery for brachial plexus birth palsy. J Bone Joint Surg Am 2007;89(1):18–26.

61. Clarke HM, Al-Qattan MM, Curtis CG, et al. Obstetrical brachial plexus palsy: results following neurolysis of conducting neuromas-in-continuity. Plast Reconstr Surg 1996;97(5):974–82 [discussion: 983-4].

62. Laurent JP, Lee R, Shenaq S, et al. Neurosurgical correction of upper brachial plexus birth injuries. J Neurosurg 1993;79(2):197–203.

63. Lin JC, Schwentker-Colizza A, Curtis CG, et al. Final results of grafting versus neurolysis in obstetrical brachial plexus palsy. Plast Reconstr Surg 2009; 123(3):939–48.

64. Xu J, Cheng X, Gu Y. Different methods and results in the treatment of obstetrical brachial plexus palsy. J Reconstr Microsurg 2000;16(6):417–20 [discussion: 420-2].

65. Manske MC, Bauer AS, Hentz VR, et al. Long-term outcomes of brachial plexus reconstruction with sural nerve autograft for brachial plexus birth injury. Plast Reconstr Surg 2019;143(5):1017e–26e.

66. Giusti G, Willems WF, Kremer T, et al. Return of motor function after segmental nerve loss in a rat model: comparison of autogenous nerve graft, collagen conduit, and processed allograft (AxoGen). J Bone Joint Surg Am 2012;94(5):410–7.

67. Garg R, Merrell GA, Hillstrom HJ, et al. Comparison of nerve transfers and nerve grafting for traumatic upper plexus palsy: a systematic review and analysis. J Bone Joint Surg Am 2011;93(9):819–29.

68. Ladak A, Morhart M, O'Grady K, et al. Distal nerve transfers are effective in treating patients with upper trunk obstetrical brachial plexus injuries: an early experience. Plast Reconstr Surg 2013;132(6):985e–92e.

69. Oberlin C, Béal D, Leechavengvongs S, et al. Nerve transfer to biceps muscle using a part of ulnar nerve for C5-C6 avulsion of the brachial plexus: anatomical study and report of four cases. J Hand Surg Am 1994;19(2):232–7.

70. Manske MC, Kalish LA, Cornwall R, et al. Reconstruction of the suprascapular nerve in brachial plexus birth injury: a comparison of nerve grafting and nerve transfers. J Bone Joint Surg Am 2020; 102(4):298–308.

71. Hinchcliff KM, Pulos N, Shin AY, et al. Morbidity of nerve transfers for brachial plexus birth injury: a systematic review. J Pediatr Orthop 2021;41(2):e188–98.

72. Davidge KM, Clarke HM, Borschel GH. Nerve transfers in birth related brachial plexus injuries: where do we stand? Hand Clin 2016;32(2):175–90.

73. Malessy MJ, Pondaag W. Neonatal brachial plexus palsy with neurotmesis of C5 and avulsion of C6: supraclavicular reconstruction strategies and outcome. J Bone Joint Surg Am 2014;96(20):e174.

74. Al-Qattan MM. Oberlin's ulnar nerve transfer to the biceps nerve in Erb's birth palsy. Plast Reconstr Surg 2002;109(1):405–7.

75. Al-Qattan MM, Al-Kharfy TM. Median nerve to biceps nerve transfer to restore elbow flexion in obstetric brachial plexus palsy. Biomed Res Int 2014; 2014:854084.

76. Little KJ, Zlotolow DA, Soldado F, et al. Early functional recovery of elbow flexion and supination following median and/or ulnar nerve fascicle transfer in upper neonatal brachial plexus palsy. J Bone Joint Surg Am 2014;96(3):215–21.

77. Siqueira MG, Socolovsky M, Heise CO, et al. Efficacy and safety of Oberlin's procedure in the treatment of brachial plexus birth palsy. Neurosurgery 2012;71(6):1156–60 [discussion: 1161].

78. Kozin SH. Nerve transfers in brachial plexus birth palsies: indications, techniques, and outcomes. Hand Clin 2008;24(4):363–76, v.

79. Dahlin LB, Erichs K, Andersson C, et al. Incidence of early posterior shoulder dislocation in brachial plexus birth palsy. J Brachial Plex Peripher Nerve Inj 2007;2:24.

80. Schmieg S, Nguyen JC, Pehnke M, et al. Team approach: management of brachial plexus birth injury. JBJS Rev 2020;8(7):e1900200.

81. Ezaki M, Malungpaishrope K, Harrison RJ, et al. Onabotulinum toxinA injection as an adjunct in the treatment of posterior shoulder subluxation in neonatal brachial plexus palsy. J Bone Joint Surg Am 2010;92(12):2171–7.

82. Troum S, Floyd WE, Waters PM. Posterior dislocation of the humeral head in infancy associated with obstetrical paralysis. A case report. J Bone Joint Surg Am 1993;75(9):1370–5.

83. Nath RK, Lyons AB, Melcher SE, et al. Surgical correction of the medial rotation contracture in obstetric brachial plexus palsy. J Bone Joint Surg Br 2007;89(12):1638–44.

84. Allard R, Fitoussi F, Azarpira MR, et al. Shoulder internal rotation contracture in brachial plexus birth injury: proximal or distal subscapularis release? J Shoulder Elbow Surg 2021;30(5):1117–27.

85. Newman CJ, Morrison L, Lynch B, et al. Outcome of subscapularis muscle release for shoulder contracture secondary to brachial plexus palsy at birth. J Pediatr Orthop 2006;26(5):647–51.

86. Jönsson K, Roos F, Hultgren T. Structures contributing to the shoulder contracture in brachial plexus birth palsy. An intraoperative biomechanical study. J Hand Surg Eur 2021. https://doi.org/10.1177/17531934211034968. 17531934211034968.

87. Waters PM, Bae DS. Effect of tendon transfers and extra-articular soft-tissue balancing on glenohumeral development in brachial plexus birth palsy. J Bone Joint Surg Am 2005;87(2):320–5.

88. Waters PM, Bae DS. The early effects of tendon transfers and open capsulorrhaphy on glenohumeral deformity in brachial plexus birth palsy. J Bone Joint Surg Am 2008;90(10):2171–9.

89. Vuillermin C, Bauer AS, Kalish LA, et al. Follow-up study on the effects of tendon transfers and open reduction on moderate glenohumeral joint deformity in brachial plexus birth injury. J Bone Joint Surg Am 2020;102(14):1260–8.

90. Waters PM, Bae DS. The effect of derotational humeral osteotomy on global shoulder function in brachial plexus birth palsy. J Bone Joint Surg Am 2006;88(5):1035–42.

91. Aly A, Bahm J, Schuind F. Percutaneous humeral derotational osteotomy in obstetrical brachial plexus palsy: a new technique. J Hand Surg Eur 2014;39(5):549–52.

92. Dodwell E, O'Callaghan J, Anthony A, et al. Combined glenoid anteversion osteotomy and tendon transfers for brachial plexus birth palsy: early outcomes. J Bone Joint Surg Am 2012;94(23):2145–52.

93. Di Mascio L, Chin KF, Fox M, et al. Glenoplasty for complex shoulder subluxation and dislocation in children with obstetric brachial plexus palsy. J Bone Joint Surg Br 2011;93(1):102–7.

94. Manske PR, McCarroll HR, Hale R. Biceps tendon rerouting and percutaneous osteoclasis in the treatment of supination deformity in obstetrical palsy. J Hand Surg Am 1980;5(2):153–9.

Peripheral Nerve Block Complications in Children

Blas Catalani, MD, MPH[a],*, Jerry Jones, Jr, MD[b,1]

KEYWORDS

- Regional anesthesia • Peripheral nerve block • Pediatric anesthesia • Complications
- Ultrasound • Local anesthetics • Intralipid • Compartment syndrome

---

KEY POINTS

- Peripheral nerve block (PNB) complications are rare in pediatric patients.
- PNBs are safely performed under general anesthesia.
- Ultrasound guidance lowers regional anesthesia complication rates and increases nerve block efficacy.
- When possible, anesthesia strategies incorporating PNBs should be selected over those using central/neuraxial techniques in pediatric patients.

INTRODUCTION

Acute pain management in children represents a significant challenge in the perioperative setting. Regional anesthesia is broadly applicable to multiple surgical disciplines and has proven to be reliable in providing postoperative analgesia and in reducing opioid utilization. Furthermore, the widespread implementation of regional anesthesia within hospital and ambulatory and nonhospital environments has become increasingly feasible over the past 20 years with the advent and incorporation of ultrasound guidance and point of care ultrasound (POCUS) technology. As with any interventional process, complications may occur, even among the most experienced anesthesiologists with formal training in ultrasound-guided regional anesthesia. This review assesses the occurrence of peripheral nerve block (PNB) complications and the underlying causes, as well as the treatment and consequences of these complications. Of note, this review will focus on peripheral regional anesthesia techniques and will only give cursory attention to other regional anesthesia techniques (central/neuraxial) for comparison purposes.

DEFINITIONS

Important distinctions regarding the terminology used to differentiate the various forms of regional anesthesia include the following:

- Neuraxial (central): local anesthetic medication injection/catheter placement in either the epidural space (outside "spinal sack") or subarachnoid/spinal space (inside the "spinal sack"). Epidural regions include caudal lumbar and thoracic. Epidural and spinal injections or infusions may include opioids.
- Peripheral: nonneuraxial injection or infusion of local anesthetic medication. May include upper and lower extremities, trunk (thoracic or abdominal regions), and/or face.
- Single shot PNB: injection of local anesthetic bolus once with or without medication adjuncts to increase the nerve block effect or duration.
- Catheter: insertion of a small hollow tube/line that is connected to an external port with the internal tip in or around the (a)

---

[a] Department of Anesthesiology, University of Tennessee HSC/College of Medicine, UTROP/Regional One Health, Memphis, TN, USA; [b] Regional Anesthesia & Acute Pain Management, Department of Anesthesiology, University of Tennessee HSC/College of Medicine, UTROP/Regional One Health, Memphis, TN, USA
[1]Present address: 5545 Murray Avenue, Suite 130, Memphis, TN 38119.
* Corresponding author. 5545 Murray Avenue, Suite 130, Memphis, TN 38119.
E-mail address: blaswork318@gmail.com

Orthop Clin N Am 53 (2022) 179–186
https://doi.org/10.1016/j.ocl.2021.11.004
0030-5898/22/© 2021 Elsevier Inc. All rights reserved.

central (epidural or subarachnoid/spinal) space or (b) peripheral nerve (perineural or within a fascial plane) space; the catheter is used for intermittent bolusing (syringe-bolus) OR connected to an infusion device (with continuous or intermittent bolusing, typically with an additional intermittent patient-demand bolus option). Note: when the catheter is inserted peripherally, this is referred to as a continuous PNB (CPNB) or peripheral nerve catheter (PNC)

- Local anesthetic systemic toxicity (LAST); a constellation of neurologic and cardiac signs or symptoms, ranging from the minor (confusion, perioral numbness or tingling, tinnitus, metallic taste) to the severe (seizure, arrhythmias, cardiac arrest) due to elevated plasma levels of local anesthetics
- Point of care ultrasound (POCUS); the use of real-time ultrasound guidance to facilitate the identification of relevant anatomic structures (eg, nerves, blood vessels, surrounding tissue elements) and to visualize the placement of regional anesthetic intervention (eg, needle-tip location, spread of local anesthetic)

COMPLICATIONS

Two large-scale, prospective, multisite, observational networks exist that have provided substantial data regarding the incidence of complications in pediatric regional anesthesia. The French Language Society of Pediatric Anaesthesiologists (ADARPEF) conducted 2 separate 12-month, prospective, multicenter, anonymous studies in Europe in 1994 and again in 2006 using 47 hospital sites. The Pediatric Regional Anesthesia Network (PRAN) was founded in 2007 and includes data on over 100,000 regional anesthetics from over 20 hospital sites in North America. These databases have been queried multiple times to facilitate many investigations, including the incidence of adverse events and complications from neuraxial and peripheral regional anesthesia techniques.

Nature of Complications

Estimating the prevalence of adverse events and/or the complications associated with performing PNBs in the pediatric population is not a precise undertaking because of the nature of the reported information. Complications from regional anesthesia are relatively rare and,

thus, require a larger sample size to be effectively evaluated. To accomplish this, data must be collected over many years to provide reliable confidence intervals, which invariably confounds data as practice patterns and available technology change through time.

Given that only 2 databases exist, and only 1 (PRAN) is continually maintained, it must be recognized that some element of reporting bias exists in the data, leading to likely underreporting of events and ultimately an underestimation of the true prevalence. Generalizing about the safety of peripheral regional anesthesia also is difficult when individual techniques have different inherent risks and are applied to patient populations that are quite diverse (eg, neonates and infants vs children >12 years old). Last, the definition and categories of complication or adverse event are interpreted differently in the 2 databases, which further complicate estimation of the true incidence. That said, the historical complication rates based on epoch data for both ADARPEF and PRAN are still valuable for the analysis of the risks of peripheral regional anesthesia in the pediatric population.

The first ADARPEF data published in 1996 included 24,409 regional anesthetics, with 89% performed under general anesthesia. Only 4090 (16%) were true PNBs and only 5.7% involved the extremities. Twenty-five complications (0.09%) occurred, but none of the complications involved PNB techniques, leading the authors to recommend at that time that PNB be selected over central techniques.[1] The second series of ADARPEF data included 31,132 patients with 96% of procedures performed under general anesthesia and 9% catheter placements (23% lower extremity, 6% upper extremity, 15% neuraxial). PNBs represented 66% of regional anesthesia techniques in this study, with 29% of PNBs for extremities. The authors identified 41 legitimate complications and determined an overall incidence of complications in pediatric regional anesthesia (combined peripheral and central) during the study window to be 0.12% (95% confidence interval (CI): 0.09–0.17). Complications were four times more frequent in children younger than 6 months of age than in children older than 6 months and seven times higher in neuraxial than peripheral techniques. Catheter use was not associated with a higher incidence of complications. For patients over 12 years of age receiving PNBs, the complication rate for PNBs was approximately six times lower than in patients receiving neuraxial/central regional anesthesia.[2]

The PRAN data reinforce this narrative of safety, indicating complications in pediatric regional anesthesia (peripheral and central techniques) to be particularly rare and estimating the risk of severe LAST to be 0.76:10,000 cases.[3] Most of these reported LAST cases occurred in infants less than 6 months of age. This is likely due to physiologic pharmacokinetic or pharmacodynamic differences in young infants rather than supratherapeutic (toxic) dosing of local anesthetic medications. The risk of superficial or cutaneous infection after regional anesthesia is estimated to be 0.5% (53:10,000 cases). There was an incidence of transient neurologic deficit of 2.4:10,000 cases, though none resulted in permanent neurologic deficits. Further, there was no additional risk observed from performing regional anesthesia under general anesthesia.[3] Anecdotal evidence of permanent neurologic injury does exist.

Other PRAN database analyses have yielded even more reassuring conclusions. One study assessing more than 40,000 PNBs (noncatheter blocks) with 93% of the blocks placed under general anesthesia found the occurrence of LAST to be 0.005% (95% CI = 0.001–0.015%).[4] This is despite the large variability in the dosing of local anesthetic medications. The PRAN data also demonstrate a substantial increase in the utilization of ultrasound-guided regional anesthesia paired with a simultaneous decrease in neurologic PNB complications, but no change in the incidence of LAST.[3]

Regarding CPNBs, the PRAN data indicate that they are safe in pediatric patients, with adverse event rates similar to adult patients. After the review of more than 2000 CPNBs, 1 study found an incidence of serious adverse complications of 0.04% (with 0 cases of LAST), an overall catheter failure rate of 1.3%, and a catheter dislodgement rate of 7.3%.[5] With regard to CPNB use for orthopaedic-specific procedures, another study examined 339 pediatric patients and found 0 cases of LAST and determined the majority of complications related to CPNB use were minor such as dislodgement or leakage (20%), temporary motor blockade (18%), nausea/vomiting (14.7%), and transient paresthesia (6.5%), indicating a high safety profile for CPNB use in pediatric patients.[6]

A concern among providers has been the safety of performing PNB or CPNB under general anesthesia. The initial ADARPEF study from 1994 found that 89% of 24,409 regional anesthetics were performed under general anesthesia, with only 5.7% being PNB of the upper or lower extremity.[1] The follow-up ADAPREF study conducted in 2006 showed a remarkable shift in pediatric regional anesthesia use with 95.9% of 29,870 regional anesthetics performed under general anesthesia, with PNB of the upper or lower extremity comprising 19.1%. The incidence of adverse postoperative neurologic symptoms in the follow-up study was 0.17%.[2] PRAN data validate these findings and further confirm the rarity of complications and the overall safety of performing regional anesthesia under general anesthesia in pediatric patients.[3,5,7]

Patient Considerations

Evaluation of the pediatric patient for placement of a PNB or CPNB involves evaluating the proposed benefits and risks presented by the anatomic and physiologic changes that occur throughout childhood as well as an assessment of the individual patient. In no way should a pediatric patient be treated as a "small adult." Additional consideration must be made for patients who have significant comorbidities (particularly cardiac, hepatic, or renal impairments). Underlying coagulopathies or history of seizures also should be identified because these may increase the risk of complications from regional anesthesia. Anatomic considerations noted in the literature reveal that the lack of age-adapted anatomic landmark techniques is a major limitation of landmark-based regional anesthesia techniques.[8] This point further emphasizes the benefits of regional anesthesia performed with real-time ultrasound guidance in appropriately trained hands.[9]

The importance of specific physiologic differences between pediatric patient populations should be considered with local anesthetic dosing, particularly patients less than 6 months of age.[10] The major physiologic considerations in this population revolve around hepatic immaturity. Specifically, reduced local anesthetic hepatic clearance associated with immature cytochrome p450 systems and the resulting increased terminal half-life of the medications lead to increased circulating concentration of free fraction of local anesthetics.

Additionally, a reduction in alpha-1-glycoprotein from hepatic immaturity leads to an increase in the free fraction of unbound local anesthetic in the plasma. This further increases the risk of LAST even with appropriate medication dosing.

From the perspective of maturity assessment and psychological preparedness, younger pediatric patients especially have difficulty tolerating minor procedures (such as peripheral IV access) and sudden movements during PNB or CPNB placement in very young patients could lead to patient injury. Because of these and other factors, regional anesthesia for pediatric patients typically is performed after the induction of general anesthesia. Accordingly, additional intraoperative time must be factored in when considering regional anesthesia for pediatric patients.

Patients and family should be educated regarding the relative risks and benefits of regional anesthesia. Appropriate management of expectations is important for maximizing postoperative recovery experiences. The need for additional education and reassurance should be anticipated with pediatric patients who may be distressed, particularly in the postoperative period if a limb cannot be moved independently or if transient paresthesia occurs during PNB resolution. Nonverbal patients present further difficulties postoperatively when evaluating pain, PNB efficacy assessment, and monitoring for minor signs and symptoms of LAST. With orthopedic surgery, intraoperative vital sign response and postoperative gross motor limb function evaluation are useful tools to evaluate appropriate PNB function.

Acute Compartment Syndrome

A recurring concern expressed regarding the use of regional anesthesia in pediatric patients (particularly trauma patients) is that of the potential to mask signs and symptoms of acute compartment syndrome (ACS). The 2018 joint publication from the American and European Societies for Regional Anesthesia and Pain Medicine (ASRA/ESRA) concluded that there is no convincing evidence that regional anesthesia complicates the diagnosis of ACS, provided patients are monitored responsibly with appropriate assessment intervals in the perioperative period[11,12] along with current best practice guidelines suggested as follows:

- Concentration of local anesthetic for a single shot in peripheral and neuraxial blocks: bupivacaine, levobupivacaine, or ropivacaine at 0.1% to 0.25% concentration. These are less likely to mask ischemic pain or to produce muscle weakness.
- Dose for continuous infusion (CPNB): bupivacaine, levobupivacaine, or ropivacaine 0.1% as the maximum permitted concentration.
- For high-risk surgery for ACS, when a sciatic nerve catheter is indicated, a restriction in LA local anesthetic volume and concentration is advisable

- Cautious use of LA local anesthetic adjuvants is recommended, as they could enhance the duration and density of the block.
- High-risk patients should be adequately evaluated by an acute pain service to allow the detection of potential, early ACS signs, and symptoms.
- If ACS is suspected, measurement of compartment pressure should be performed urgently.

Selection of Local Anesthetic Medications

In pediatric patients, proper selection and accurate dosing of local anesthetic medications are paramount to successful perioperative and postoperative management goals. Amide-class local anesthetics are preferred over ester-local anesthetics for their reduced incidence of allergic reactions, greater lipid solubility and potency, prolonged duration of action, and a greater stability to hydrolysis.[1] Ropivacaine and levobupivacaine are the drugs of choice in pediatric regional anesthesia, owing to their safer cardiac and neurotoxicity profiles (reduced risk of LAST) with ropivacaine having an increased motor-sparing effect. Dosing recommendations per ASRA/ESRA recommendations[11,12] for extremity (upper and lower) PNBs is 0.5 to 1.5 mL/kg using either ropivacaine 0.2%, levobupivacaine 0.25%, or bupivacaine 0.25%.[12]

MANAGEMENT OF COMPLICATIONS

Nonpharmacological Intervention

The rarest of circumstances with PNB/CPNB might require surgical intervention. This is largely reserved for significant malfunctions in equipment, such as a broken needle or retained catheter that must be surgically retrieved, or incision and drainage for superficial infection when conservative measures fail. Otherwise, major surgery is relegated to complications of central/neuraxial anesthesia (eg, abscess or hematoma evacuation).

As for cutaneous reactions, these are largely minor (eg, minor erythema, induration, or inflammation) and are best managed initially with conservative methods (ice application, observation). In the unlikely event of progression, escalation of care may be indicated.

Pharmacologic Intervention

In the event of a cutaneous infection resulting from a PNB or CPNB, proposed antibiotic therapy (when indicated) should be guided by resulting laboratory information. Empiric antibiotic therapy is not routinely required.

Also very uncommon, yet substantially more severe are major signs and symptoms of LAST. The method of LAST treatment depends on whether symptoms are minor or major as well as the rapidity of symptom escalation. Many of the signs and symptoms of LAST may be masked in the pediatric population by general anesthesia and the use of intraoperative muscle relaxants. Successful management of major symptoms of LAST depends entirely on close and ongoing patient evaluation and early initiation of lipid resuscitation therapy (LRT) using Intralipid 20% emulsion when the diagnosis is suspected or confirmed. Minor LAST symptomology is usually self-limited. Conservative treatment in this circumstance involves cessation of PNB local anesthetic injection or CPNB infusion (with subsequent rate or medication adjustments), supplemental oxygen, and ensuring that intravenous (IV) access and emergency equipment and supplies are available. The patient and family should be reassured, and patients should be monitored until symptoms are resolved. If minor symptoms are ongoing or escalating, benzodiazepines are appropriate to avoid neurologic symptoms such as seizures. In the event that minor symptoms represent heralding findings with progression to severe LAST and associated neuro or cardiac toxicity, initiation of LRT with Intralipid in accordance with the recommendations of the Society for Pediatric Anesthesia Checklist should be initiated:[11,13]

- Stop injecting the local anesthetic and call for help and intralipid kit.
- Confirm or establish adequate IV access.
- Maintain the airway and give 100% oxygen. Consider the placement of endotracheal tube.
- Continuously monitor electrocardiogram (ECG), blood pressure (BP), oxygen saturation by pulse oximetry (SpO2).
- If seizures develop, administer a benzodiazepine (eg, midazolam 0.05–0.1 mg/kg/min IV), watch resultant hypotension.
- Avoid routine advanced cardiac life support (ACLS) doses of epinephrine. Treat hypotension with small IV epinephrine dose (MAX: 1mcg/kg)
- *Drugs to Avoid:* propofol, vasopressin, calcium channel blockers, and beta-blockers.
- Start IV intralipid therapy as follows:
  - Initial bolus: IV 20% lipid emulsion = 1.5 mL/kg over 60 seconds

  - Maintenance infusion: IV 20% lipid emulsion = 0.25 mL/kg/min
  - Repeat IV bolus every 3 to 5 min until circulation is restored
    - MAX cumulative total bolus dosing = 4.5 mL/kg
  - If cardiovascular instability persists, double infusion rate to 0.5 mL/kg/min
    - Continue maintenance infusion for 10 mins once hemodynamic stability is restored
  - Note: total intralipid dose should not exceed 10 mL/kg
- Recognize arrhythmias and/or cardiac arrest and initiate cardiopulmonary resuscitation (CPR)/pediatric advanced life support (PALS) protocols
  - *REMEMBER:* Continue chest compressions as intralipid must circulate to be effective
    - May need prolonged compressions
- *6-min mark:* Consider alerting nearest cardiopulmonary bypass or extracorporeal membrane oxygenation (ECMO) center and intensive care unit if there is no return to spontaneous circulation to facilitate the transfer and maintenance of circulation until local anesthetic is metabolized.
- Monitor and correct acidosis, hypercarbia, and hyperkalemia as needed.

Prevention of Complications

Although the treatment of regional anesthesia complications generally is very successful, there are several processes that will limit or mitigate complications associated with peripheral regional anesthesia if used routinely. Regarding the prevention of infection or adverse cutaneous findings, the injection site should be thoroughly cleansed with a chlorhexidine or similar substance to ensure the aseptic (PNB) or sterile (CPNB) integrity of the procedure. CPNB dressings and catheter sites should be monitored routinely along with other general signs and symptoms of infection. Disconnecting or opening CPNB catheters to air should be kept to a minimum.

Preventing neurologic injury from needle trauma involves the use of real-time ultrasound guidance to avoid needle-to-nerve contact or use fascial "plane approaches" and instead favor perineural injections whenever possible. Injections of a local anesthetic should be performed with low pressure and intermittent bolusing.

As previously discussed, using precise local anesthetic dose calculations, taking into account physiologic reasons that may predispose individual patients to LAST is essential. Further, injections of local anesthetic should be incremental, and local anesthetics should be visualized with real-time ultrasound guidance for appropriate spread and followed by intermittent aspirations between boluses to ensure intravascular placement has not occurred. Finally, continuous vital-sign monitoring should occur during and after local anesthetic injections.

DISCUSSION

The use of PNB or CPNB to facilitate perioperative anesthetic and analgesic goals for pediatric patients has proliferated significantly in recent years. In many regions, data show an inversion of trends that reflect preferential selection of peripheral over central regional anesthesia techniques.[14] This trend can be attributed largely to the recognized safety and reliability of ultrasound-guided peripheral regional anesthesia in the pediatric population especially when compared with central/neuraxial techniques, new and more refined PNB approaches and techniques, and the availability of LRT/lipid emulsion 20% for the treatment of LAST.

The biggest limitation to the assessment of the safety profiles and complication rates related to PNB and CPNB in pediatric patients relate to the sources of available data. The aggregate data from the PRAN and ADARPEF studies includes both central/neuraxial and peripheral categories of regional anesthetics, and the published conclusions drawn from this aggregated data regarding complications were derived with both central and peripheral techniques in mind. These studies, however, do indicate that central regional anesthesia and minor CPNB catheter-related issues account for the vast majority of complications. This makes the true estimation of isolated peripheral nerve PNB and CPNB complication rates (prevalence and incidence) difficult to determine, although it is likely lower than the resulting published overall incidence rates for regional anesthesia complications in pediatric populations.

The ethical and practical considerations of performing PNB techniques for perioperative anesthetic and analgesic management are well defined. A postoperative course without significant pain or reliance on opioids raises the morale of the patient, parents, medical staff, and surgical team, and it is not justifiable to allow a pediatric patient to suffer pain when reliable and safe regional anesthesia techniques are available.[15] Regional anesthesia, and, in particular, PNB techniques, complement existing management strategies, and facilitate a comprehensively safer experience for the pediatric patient, but also ultimately cultivates a more satisfactory experience for all involved.

SUMMARY

Complications associated with PNB and CPNB regional anesthesia techniques include:

- Nerve block failure or incomplete nerve block coverage
- Patient   anxiety/psychological traumatization
- Neurologic:
  - Minor neurologic symptoms
  - Seizures
  - Nerve damage (needle, chemical-induced)
  - Transient paresthesia
  - Prolonged motor block
- Cardiovascular:
  - Minor or major arrhythmias
  - Cardiac arrest
  - Inadvertent vascular puncture
  - Minor or major vascular injury with bleeding or hematoma formation
- Cutaneous and superficial infection (rare)
- CPNB dislodgement/disconnection or mechanical failure
- Potential to mask ACS
- Upper extremity blocks
  - Phrenic palsy (hemidiaphragm) with respiratory distress
  - Pneumothorax
  - Horner's syndrome (temporary)
- Lower extremity blocks
  - Fall Risk

CLINICAL CARE POINTS

Evidence-based pearls
- Ultrasound guidance:
  - Lowers complications[3]
  - Decreases risk of LAST[16]
  - Increases effective duration of PNB and decreases postoperative pain scores[17]
- PNB/CPNB/regional anesthesia:
  - Safe to be performed after the induction of general anesthesia[2,3]

- o Placement under general anesthesia should be considered the standard technique in children[11]
- • Anesthetic and analgesia strategy:
  - o Strategies including PNB/CPNB use should be selected over those involving central/neuraxial regional anesthetic use in pediatric patients (when possible) due to reduced morbidity[2]
- • PNBs do not mask ACS findings in the proper care settings[11]

Pitfalls relevant to the point of care

The majority of the challenges presented to the care team related to the implementation of regional anesthesia in the pediatric population, particularly PNB techniques, are related to 2 items: patient selection and management infrastructure.

- • Pediatric patients are difficult to assess for both chief complaint, block efficacy, and possible signs of toxic local anesthetic dosing; this is particularly relevant in preverbal/nonverbal children
- • Regimen compliance is generally more difficult to ensure (especially with variable/unpredictable support systems/guardians)
- • Without adequate patient/guardian education (especially in the ambulatory care setting) and absence of routine and comprehensive follow-up with patients, adverse events and preventable complications will occur. Most important of all is the requirement to incorporate a properly trained and educated anesthesiology care team to ensure that the use of regional anesthesia and PNB techniques results in the highest quality results with consistent patient safety and satisfaction outcomes.

DISCLOSURE

B. Catalani has nothing to disclose. J. Jones has a financial relationship (Founder, Patent Holder, Major Stock Owner) with Cal Tenn Innovations Inc., a company designing a medical device for use in ultrasound imaging. He has consulted for numerous medical devices companies related to nerve block devices, but none in the past 12 months. The content of this manuscript has not been influenced by these factors or by any commercial entity.

REFERENCES

1. Giaufré E, Dalens B, Gombert A. Epidemiology and morbidity of regional anesthesia in children: a one-year prospective survey of the French-Language Society of Pediatric Anesthesiologists. Anesth Analg 1996;83(5):904–12.

2. Ecoffey C, Lacroix F, Giaufré E, et al. Association des Anesthésistes Réanimateurs Pédiatriques d'Expression Française (ADARPEF). Epidemiology and morbidity of regional anesthesia in children: a follow-up one-year prospective survey of the French-Language Society of Paediatric Anaesthesiologists (ADARPEF). Paediatr Anaesth 2010;20(12):1061–9.

3. Walker BJ, Long JB, Sathyamoorthy M, et al. Complications in pediatric regional anesthesia: an analysis of more than 100,000 blocks from the pediatric regional anesthesia network. Anesthesiology 2018;129(4):721–32.

4. Suresh S, De Oliveira GS Jr. Local anaesthetic dosage of peripheral nerve blocks in children: analysis of 40121 blocks from the Pediatric Regional Anesthesia Network database. Br J Anaesth 2018;120(2):317–22 [Erratum in: Br J Anaesth 2018;121(3):686].

5. Walker BJ, De Oliveira GS, Szmuk P, et al. Peripheral nerve catheters in children: an analysis of safety and practice patterns from the Pediatric Regional Anesthesia Network (PRAN). Br J Anaesth 2015;115(3):457–62.

6. Dadure C, Bringuier S, Raux O, et al. Continuous peripheral nerve blocks for postoperative analgesia in children: feasibility and side effects in a cohort study of 339 catheters. Can J Anaesth 2009;56(11):843–50.

7. Polaner DM, Taenzer AH, Walker BJ, et al. Pediatric Regional Anesthesia Network (PRAN): a multi-institutional study of the use and incidence of complications of pediatric regional anesthesia. Anesth Analg 2012;115(6):1353–64.

8. Byun S, Pather N. Pediatric regional anesthesia: A review of the relevance of surface anatomy and landmarks used for peripheral nerve blockades in infants and children. Clin Anat 2019;32(6):803–23.

9. Marhofer P. Upper extremity peripheral blocks. Tech Reg Anesth Pain Manag 2007;11:215–21.

10. Heydinger G, Tobias J, Veneziano G. Fundamentals and innovations in regional anaesthesia for infants and children. Anaesthesia 2021;76(Suppl 1):74–88.

11. Merella F, Canchi-Murali N, Mossetti V. General principles of regional anaesthesia in children. BJA Educ 2019;19(10):342–8 [Erratum in: BJA Educ 2020 Jan;20(1):32].

12. Suresh S, Ecoffey C, Bosenberg A, et al. The European Society of Regional Anaesthesia and Pain Therapy/American Society of Regional Anesthesia and Pain Medicine recommendations on local anesthetics and adjuvants dosage in pediatric regional anesthesia. Reg Anesth Pain Med 2018;43(2):211–6.

13. Society for Pediatric Anesthesia. Pedi Critical Events Checklists. Section 17: Local Anesthetic Toxicity. 2018. Available at: https://www.pedsanesthesia.org/wp- content/uploads/2018/11/SPAPediCrisisChecklists Nov2018.pdf. Accessed September 22, 2021.

14. Vicchio N, Mossetti V, Ivani G. Evaluation of 18279 blocks in a pediatric hospital. Anesth Pain Med 2015;5(2):e22897.

15. Simić D, Stević M, Stanković Z, et al. The safety and efficacy of the continuous peripheral nerve block in postoperative analgesia of pediatric patients. Front Med (Lausanne) 2018;5:57.

16. Barrington MJ, Kluger R. Ultrasound guidance reduces the risk of local anesthetic systemic toxicity following peripheral nerve blockade. Reg Anesth Pain Med 2013;38(4):289–99.

17. Guay J, Suresh S, Kopp S. The use of ultrasound guidance for perioperative neuraxial and peripheral nerve blocks in children. Cochrane Database Syst Rev 2019;2(2):CD011436.

Hand and Wrist

Digital Nerve Reconstruction

Thomas R. Acott, MD

KEYWORDS

- Digital nerve reconstruction • Conduit repair • Autograft nerve reconstruction
- Allograft nerve reconstruction • Digital nerve gap

KEY POINTS

- If primary end-to-end neurorrhaphy is not possible because of a nerve gap after adequate debridement of nerve ends, a nerve reconstruction should be performed.
- Options include conduit repair, autograft reconstruction, and allograft reconstruction.
- Multiple comparison studies exist, suggesting similar results with autograft and allograft reconstruction, with several studies suggesting inferior outcomes with conduit repair.

INTRODUCTION

Nerve injuries are commonly encountered by hand and upper extremity surgeons, with 81% of peripheral nerve injuries occurring in the upper extremity[1] and most commonly involving the digital nerves.[2] Digital nerve injuries may lead to numbness and sensory loss, digital and hand impairment, pain, cold intolerance, hyperesthesia, and decreased quality of life. Timely and appropriate treatment can optimize patient outcomes.

The goal of surgical treatment is primary end-to-end neurorrhaphy. However, primary repair is not always possible because of a wide zone of injury or retraction of nerve ends, both of which create a nerve defect. More research is being conducted on the management of digital nerve defects. Recent series on nerve reconstruction have demonstrated improved sensory recovery compared with older series,[3] likely due to increased research and awareness and improved technical ability to handle intraoperative nerve defects. This article aims to review current literature on digital nerve reconstruction and the management of digital nerve defects.

EVALUATION

Mechanisms of injury to a digital nerve may include sharp lacerations, punctures, as well as saw, crush, avulsion, or gunshot injuries. Patients often provide a history of altered or decreased sensation in the affected nerve distribution. A detailed history should be obtained, noting medical comorbidities (including diabetes, immunocompromised states, peripheral neuropathy, etc) that may affect patient outcomes, as well as handedness, occupation, and recreational hobbies.

Patients should be evaluated for concomitant injuries involving tendons, digital arteries, fractures, as well as the condition of the overlying soft-tissue envelope.[4] Concomitant injuries have been reported to occur in up to 56% to 76% of digital nerve injuries.[5,6]

Neurologic examination includes sensory, motor, pain, electrodiagnostic, and patient-reported outcome measures.[1] Sensory outcome measures are often used to compare treatment outcomes. Sensation to light touch in the affected nerve distribution is often abnormal, but this is subjective and therefore not often cited in the literature.

Sensory examination includes 2-point discrimination (static and moving) and Semmes-Weinstein (SW) monofilament testing. Two-point discrimination assesses the tactile gnosis or the ability of the hand to recognize objects or textures.[1] Static 2-point discrimination assesses the innervation density of slowly adapting receptors that continually fire when pressure is applied, whereas moving 2-point

The CORE Institute, 18444 North 25th Avenue, Suite. 210, Phoenix, AZ 85023, USA
E-mail address: thomas.acott@thecoreinstitute.com

Orthop Clin N Am 53 (2022) 187–195
https://doi.org/10.1016/j.ocl.2021.12.003
0030-5898/22/© 2021 Elsevier Inc. All rights reserved.

discrimination assesses quickly adapting receptors that fire at the onset and offset of stimulation.[1] Two-point discrimination is often cited in the literature (Table 1), but because of a lack of performance standardization, it is not recommended as the only assessment of sensory recovery.[1] This variability in technique raises concerns when comparing 2-point discrimination sensory outcomes in the literature. SW monofilament testing quantitatively assesses the cutaneous pressure threshold.[1] The modified British Medical Research Council (BMRC) score combines subjective findings and 2-point discrimination and is often used as an outcome measure in the literature[1] (Table 2).

Pain and patient-reported outcomes are assessed using the visual analog scale (VAS), 36-Item Short Form Health Survey (SF-36), Disabilities of the Arm, Shoulder and Hand (DASH), and Michigan Hand Outcomes Questionnaire (MHQ). Cold sensitivity may be assessed using the Cold Sensitivity Severity Scale.[1] Electrodiagnostic studies are less commonly performed for digital nerves than mixed-motor and motor nerves.

NONOPERATIVE TREATMENT

Nonoperative treatment of a digital nerve injury may be pursued in accordance with the patient's values and wishes or it may be a result of neglect or a missed diagnosis. Untreated digital nerve injuries result in sensory loss and may impair fine motor skills and proprioception.[2] It may also put the digit at risk for further injury.[2] Axonal sprouting can disperse, leading to neuroma formation, which may result in pain and further functional impairment.[7] Cold sensitivity, which may present as pain, numbness, stiffness, swelling, or change in skin color, may also result.[1]

OPERATIVE TREATMENT

The goal of surgical treatment of a nerve injury is primary end-to-end repair. A successful nerve

Table 2	
British Medical Research Council Sensory Scale, modified by Mackinnon and Dellon	
	British Medical Research Council Sensory Scale[1,2]
S0	Absence of sensibility in the autonomous area of the nerve
S1	Recovery of deep cutaneous pain and tactile sensibility
S2	Recovery of some degree of superficial cutaneous pain and tactile sensibility
S3	Return of superficial cutaneous pain and tactile sensibility with disappearance of overresponse; S2PD >15 mm, M2PD >7 mm
S3+	Return of sensibility as in S3 with some recovery of 2-point discrimination; S2PD: 7–15 mm, M2PD: 4–7 mm
S4	Complete recovery; S2PD: 2–6 mm, M2PD: 2–3 mm

repair involves adequate resection of nerve ends, delicate handling of the nerve and soft tissues, and tension-free repair in a well-vascularized wound bed.[8,9] The nerve ends should be resected until healthy nerve substance ("sprouting fascicles") are encountered. A wide zone of injury that creates damaged nerve ends, particularly in injuries involving crush or avulsion mechanisms, or delayed repair associated with excessive nerve scarring or retraction, may result in a nerve gap after adequate resection. Following nerve-end debridement, the nerve should be assessed for a defect with the digits extended.[10] When a nerve defect precludes tensionless primary end-to-end repair,[2,9] a nerve reconstruction should instead be performed. Nerve reconstruction is preferred to primary neurorrhaphy with inadequate resection of nerve ends, or end-to-end nerve repair requiring tension after adequate nerve-end debridement.[9]

Nerve tension has a negative effect on peripheral nerve regeneration. Animal studies have shown that eliminating tension at the repair site improves nerve regeneration.[11] This is due to several mechanisms. Tension has been shown to affect nerve perfusion, with elongation of greater than 15% leading to a substantial and irreversible reduction in blood flow.[12,13] Tension also impairs Schwann cell activation and induces

Table 1	
Outcomes for static 2-point discrimination	
Grade	**S2PD (mm)**
Excellent	<6
Good	6–10
Fair	11–15
Poor	>15 or protective sensation

Schwann cell apoptosis, with a negative effect on axonal outgrowth.[14] Mechanical failure also may occur with elongation of 16% to 17%.[12]

Several options exist to deal with resultant nerve defects, including conduit repair and nerve reconstruction with nerve autograft or allograft.

CONDUIT

Conduits are hollow semirigid tubes (**Fig. 1**). They function by serving as a guide for sprouting axons, providing a barrier against ingrowth of scar tissue, and maintaining an internal environment for nerve regeneration.[7,15] Although autologous sources (most commonly vein) may be used, conduits are often manufactured and most commonly composed of polyglycolic acid (PGA), collagen, or poly (DL-lactide-ε-caprolactone).[9,16] Conduits resist collapse and kinking and are semipermeable, allowing passage of oxygen and nutrients to support nerve regeneration while maintaining an increased concentration of fibrin and nerve growth factors that are secreted by damaged nerve ends.[15–17] Some conduits degrade with time after nerve regeneration.[9,16] An advantage is the lack of donor site morbidity. It has been suggested that surgeons may be more willing to adequately debride nerve endings when conduits are available to repair the resultant nerve gap.[3,18]

An appropriately sized conduit is first selected. The nerve ends are drawn into the conduit 3 to 5mm and secured with 8-0 or 9-0 horizontal mattress suture[15,17,19,20] (**Fig. 2**). The conduit is often injected with saline, heparinized saline, or lactated Ringer solution[15,18–20](**Fig. 3**).

Multiple series have investigated bovine collagen conduits (NeuraGen Nerve Guide, Integra LifeSciences Corporation, Cincinnati, OH, USA). In their series, Taras and colleagues included gaps less than 20 mm (average defect 12 mm) and found that all patients recovered protective sensation with moving 2-point discrimination of 5 mm and static 2-point discrimination of 5 mm. They found an excellent result in 59%, good result in 14%, fair result in 27%, and no poor results.[15] Haug and colleagues assessed collagen conduits for 5 to 26 mm defects (average 12 mm) and found very good or good recovery in 60% of repairs. Age less than 50 years and distance to end organ 50 mm or less also positively affected outcomes, whereas circular saws and iatrogenic injuries negatively affected outcomes.[17] Bushnell and colleagues performed conduit repairs for defects 1 to 2 cm and found excellent or good results in 89%, with 11% fair results.[21] In a series investigating bioabsorbable PGA conduits, Mackinnon and colleagues found excellent outcomes in 33%, good outcomes in 53%, with 14% rated as treatment failures when used for gaps 5 to 30 mm (average 17 mm).[19] Conduits have been shown to be safe, with multiple series reporting no complications related to conduit use.[15,21] Silicone conduits have been abandoned because of concern over foreign body reactions and irritation.[22]

Reversed autologous veins from the dorsal hand or volar forearm may be used.

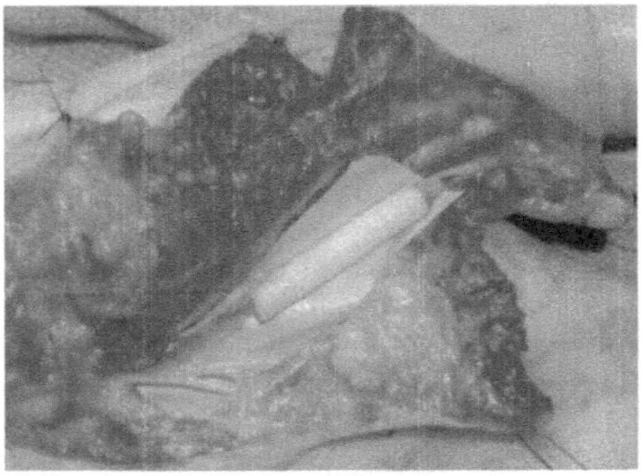

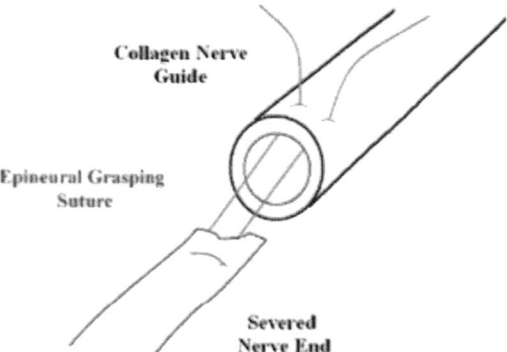

Fig. 1. Completed repair. View of a collagen nerve tube used to repair a gap defect in a digital nerve of the left thumb. (Reproduced from Bushnell BD, McWilliams AD, Whitener GB, Messer TM. Early clinical experience with collagen nerve tubes in digital nerve repair. J Hand Surg Am. 2008;33(7):1081-1087. https://doi.org/10.1016/j.jhsa.2008.03.015.)

Fig. 2. Suturing the nerve end into the collagen nerve tube. An epineural grasping suture is used to pull the severed end of the injured nerve into the nerve tube and secure it in place. (Reproduced from Bushnell BD, McWilliams AD, Whitener GB, Messer TM. Early clinical experience with collagen nerve tubes in digital nerve repair. J Hand Surg Am. 2008;33(7):1081-1087. https://doi.org/10.1016/j.jhsa.2008.03.015.)

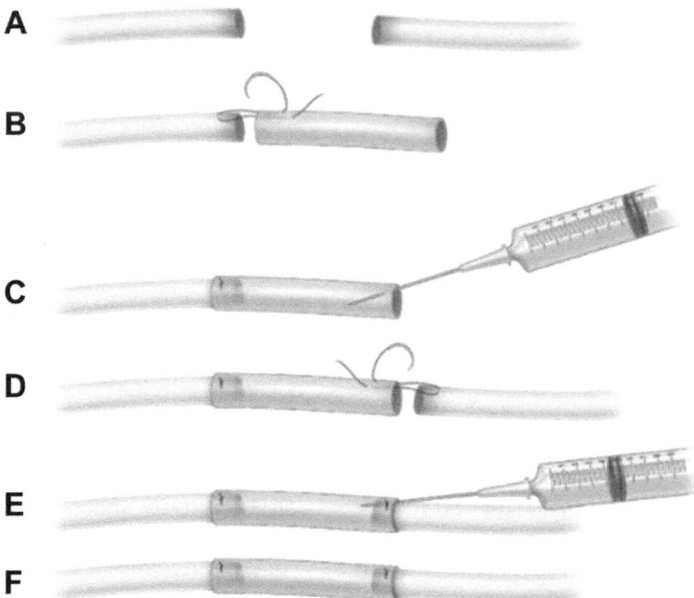

Fig. 3. Schematic of collagen conduit technique. (A) Injured nerve ends are isolated and trimmed. (B) Epineurium is sutured to the conduit using an 8-0 monofilament, nonabsorbable suture. (C) The lumen of the conduit is filled with saline to prevent a clot from forming within it. (D) The other injured nerve end is sutured in the same fashion as the first end. (E) Final filling of the conduit lumen with saline. (F) Final appearance after repair with a conduit. (Printed with permission of Integra LifeSciences Corporation, Plainsboro, NJ.) (Reproduced from Taras JS, Jacoby SM, Lincoski CJ. Reconstruction of digital nerves with collagen conduits. J Hand Surg Am. 2011;36(9):1441-1446. https://doi.org/10.1016/j.jhsa.2011.06.009.)

Disadvantages of vein conduits include additional surgical time, donor site complications, and collapse of the vein conduit that may affect nerve regrowth.[3,20]

PGA conduits have shown similar results (static and moving 2-point discrimination) at 1 year as compared to autogenous vein conduits. PGA conduits were found to have a shorter surgical time, with no difference, however, in total cost.[20] Short gaps had greater recovery than long gaps (>10 mm), and smokers and workman's compensation had worse sensory recovery. Although complication rates did not reach significance, there were 2 PGA conduit extrusions that required reoperation.[20]

AUTOGRAFT

Autograft reconstruction involves harvesting an autologous sensory nerve to repair a digital nerve. Common sources include sural nerve, medial antebrachial cutaneous nerve (MABCN), lateral antebrachial cutaneous nerve (LABCN), and the posterior interosseous nerve (PIN). The ideal donor nerve should be easy to harvest, provide sufficient length, be constant in its anatomic location, and have minimal donor-site morbidity.[4] Disadvantages of autograft are related to donor-site morbidity including sensory loss, neuroma, and scar formation, as well as the additional surgical time and cost of harvest.[3,23] Up to 20% to 30% of patients may experience pain related to the donor site.[9]

Stang and colleagues compared PIN versus MABCN autograft for average 22-mm defects. They found no difference in sensory outcomes but recommended use of the PIN because of the easier donor harvest and decreased donor site morbidity. Two to 3 cm of the PIN may be harvested proximal to the fourth dorsal compartment, deep to the extensor digitorum communis and extensor indicis proprius. The only reported morbidity was the visible scar on the dorsal wrist. The authors harvested the anterior branch of the MABCN 3 cm distal to the medial epicondyle, avoiding harvest of the posterior branch that results in numbness over the olecranon. Most patients complained about the resultant scar and unpleasant paresthesias that occurred when resting the forearm on a desk. The area of sensory loss measured 16 × 8 cm. In addition, 25% had painful neuromas. However, the MABCN may still have a role in more extensive injuries because of the MABCN's additional length and arborization.[4]

The LABCN graft may be harvested from the proximal third of the lateral forearm, roughly 6 to 7 cm distal to antecubital flexion crease. Using static 2-point discrimination, Pilanci and colleagues reported 33% excellent results, 53% good results, and 13% moderate results with an average LABCN harvest of 18 mm. Using the BMRC, they reported 100% ≥S3+ recovery. All patients reported anterolateral forearm numbness, but this was not bothersome and likely caused by the area of numbness not being on the resting surface of the forearm. Thirteen percent did report cold intolerance at the donor site; no neuromas were reported.[22] The sensory deficit created by harvest of the LABCN overlaps with the superficial branch of the radial nerve in 75% of patients, helping to minimize the sensory deficit.[24]

Up to 30 to 40 cm of sural nerve may be harvested for nerve graft.[24] Sural nerve may be harvested using a longitudinal approach, or multiple transverse incisions with a more cosmetic scar.[24] IJpma and colleagues reported long-term results (average 26-year follow-up) of sural nerve harvest morbidity. The authors buried the proximal sural nerve stump into muscle after harvest. They reported a 5 × 6 cm area of sensory loss in the sural nerve distribution over the posterolateral distal leg and lateral ankle, heel, and foot. Significant improvement in sensory loss, pain, and cold sensitivity was noted to occur up to 5 years after harvest, at which time it plateaued. This was attributed to collateral sprouting and regeneration from adjacent intact sensory nerves that help reinnervate the affected area, in addition to cortical remapping in which adjacent intact nerves are remapped to the cortical area previously occupied by the harvested donor nerve. Despite this improvement over the first 5 years, 20% to 30% of patients still experienced pain, cold sensitivity, scar discomfort, and functional impairment, reported mostly with direct contact and when putting on shoes. Fourteen percent of patients were not satisfied with their outcome involving the donor site.[25]

Higgins and colleagues performed a cadaver study investigating various donor nerves for digital reconstruction[24] (Figs. 4 and 5). The sural nerve was found to be the most similar graft for common digital nerve defects based on cross-sectional area and number of fascicles, with the sural nerve being smaller with fewer fascicles than the common digital nerve (Figs. 6 and 7). The LABCN was the best match for proper digital nerve defects (proximal to the distal trifurcation); however, the LABCN was also found to have significantly fewer fascicles than the proper digital nerve[24](Table 3).

ALLOGRAFT

Processed human nerve allograft was developed as an alternative to autograft to avoid the donor site morbidity and additional surgical time associated with autograft.[10,16] These became commercially available in the United States in 2007.[5] The grafts are decellularized and irradiated while preserving the 3-dimensional extracellular matrix and laminin-rich endoneurial tubes, which support axonal regeneration.[9,10] The presence of extracellular matrix distinguishes allografts from conduits. The

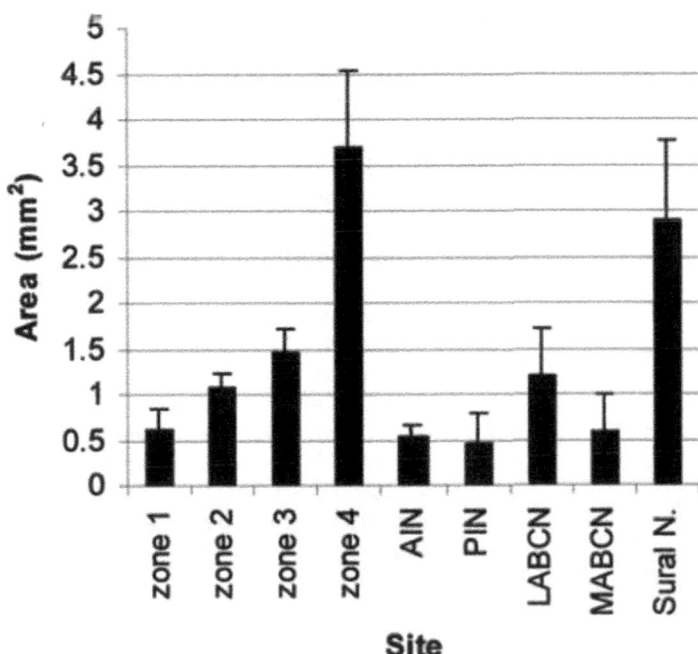

Fig. 4. Mean cross-sectional area of all sample sites with SD. (Reproduced from Higgins JP, Fisher S, Serletti JM, Orlando GS. Assessment of nerve graft donor sites used for reconstruction of traumatic digital nerve defects. J Hand Surg Am. 2002;27(2):286-292. https://doi.org/10.1053/jhsu.2002.)

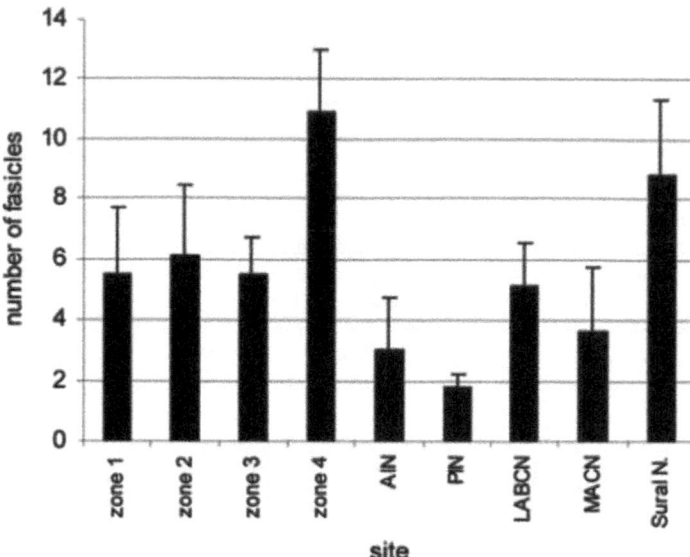

Fig. 5. Mean number of fascicles of all sample sites with SD. (Reproduced from Higgins JP, Fisher S, Serletti JM, Orlando GS. Assessment of nerve graft donor sites used for reconstruction of traumatic digital nerve defects. J Hand Surg Am. 2002;27(2):286-292. https://doi.org/10.1053/jhsu.2002.)

decellularization avoids the need for immune suppression; however, the risk of infectious disease transmission remains.[3,16,23]

The RANGER Study, a multicenter registry created in 2007 and funded by AxoGen, Inc, has investigated the use of Avance Nerve Graft (AxoGen Inc, Alachua, FL, USA), with multiple published series. In an early series, Cho and colleagues studied the use in digital nerve, mixed-motor, and motor nerves with an average defect of 22 mm. They found sensory recovery of ≥S3 (meaningful level of recovery) in 89% of digital nerve repairs without reported complications.[26] In a series investigating allograft

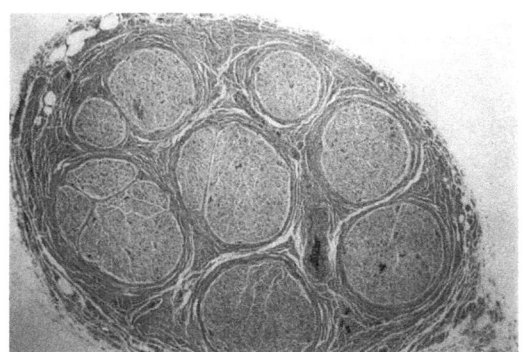

Fig. 6. Zone 4 digital nerve (hematoxylin-eosin, original magnification ×2). (Reproduced from Higgins JP, Fisher S, Serletti JM, Orlando GS. Assessment of nerve graft donor sites used for reconstruction of traumatic digital nerve defects. J Hand Surg Am. 2002;27(2):286-292. https://doi.org/10.1053/jhsu.2002.)

use in short defects (average 11 mm), Rinker and colleagues found meaningful recovery (≥S3-S4) in 92% of repairs, with ≥S3+ in 84% of repairs. They reported average static 2-point discrimination of 7 mm, average moving 2-point discrimination of 6 mm, and return of protective sensation or greater in 88%, with 72% reporting return to light touch using SW monofilament.[5] In another series investigating use in large nerve defects (>25 mm defects, average 35 mm), Rinker and colleagues reported ≥ S3 sensory recovery in 86%. Their reported sensory recovery was consistent across gap lengths, with 89% recovery for gaps 26 to 39 mm, and 86% for gaps 40 to 50 mm. The average static 2-point discrimination was 9 mm, with 87% recovering protective sensation.[8] The authors of these series reported that their results are comparable with historical reports using autograft, and exceed results for conduits.[5,8,26] In a non-RANGER series (but supported by AxoGen, Inc), Taras and colleagues reported 83% good/excellent results for defects up to 30 mm (average 11 mm). They reported average static 2-point discrimination of 7 mm, average moving 2-point discrimination of 5 mm, with improvements in VAS and QuickDASH scores.[10] Allograft has been reported to be safe without complications.[5,10,26]

COMPARISON STUDIES

Two studies (both supported by AxoGen Inc) have compared conduit repair to allograft

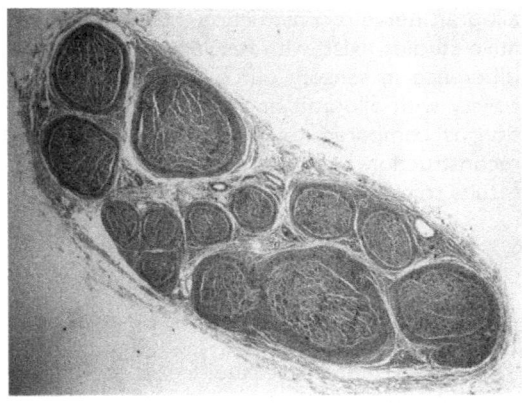

Fig. 7. Sural nerve (hematoxylin-eosin, original magnification ×2). (Reproduced from Higgins JP, Fisher S, Serletti JM, Orlando GS. Assessment of nerve graft donor sites used for reconstruction of traumatic digital nerve defects. J Hand Surg Am. 2002;27(2):286-292. https://doi.org/10.1053/jhsu.2002.)

reconstruction and have found allografts to be superior. Leversedge and colleagues found allograft reconstructions to have statistically higher rates of meaningful recovery (88% allograft, 61% conduit) in 13 to 14 mm defects. They found significantly better return of static 2-point discrimination in the allograft group (allograft 9 mm, conduit 12 mm). Similar recovery was reported in the allograft group in short and long defects; however, the conduit group was noted to have decreased recovery with increasing gap length. The conduit group had a higher rate of neuroma formation (12% vs 3%), whereas the allograft group did have one infection.[9] In a randomized double-blinded study, allograft reconstruction was found to have significantly better and more consistent sensory recovery as compared with conduits. All allograft reconstructions had return of static 2-point discrimination, versus only 75% of conduits, with an average static 2-point discrimination of 5 mm (allograft) versus 8 mm (conduit). All allograft reconstructions were found to have S3+ recovery and 83% had S4 recovery, whereas in the conduit group only 75% recovered S3+ and 50% had S4 recovery. Both techniques were successful in preventing neuromas.[7]

Two systemic reviews found similar sensory recovery between autograft and allograft reconstructions, with both being superior to conduit reconstruction.[2,23] One systemic review found similar static 2-point discrimination and SW monofilament sensory outcomes in autograft and allograft reconstruction, with inferior outcomes seen with conduit use. Average gap sizes reported were allograft 15 mm, autograft 25 mm, and conduit 13 mm.[23] Another systemic review found a higher percentage of normal or near normal recovery in autograft and allograft reconstruction, with conduits demonstrating a higher rate of incomplete sensory recovery and increased complications. Average defects reported were autograft 22 mm, allograft 13 mm, and conduit 12 mm. In 88% of autografts, 86% of allograft, and 77% of conduit reconstructions, ≥S3+ recovery was reported. Similarly, they found return of static 2-point discrimination in 100% of allograft, 88% of autograft, and 72% of conduits. Normal or diminished light touch with SW was reported in 93% after autograft, 71% after allograft, and 46% after conduits. Contrary to other studies, they found conduits to have a higher complication rate (10.9%) than autograft (5.7%) and allograft (3.0%). Complication types were different; all autograft complications were MABCN neuromas, all allograft complications were infections, and conduit complications included infection, extrusion, amputation, or removal. The authors concluded that conduits are best used for shorter gaps and less complex injuries.[2]

Other systemic reviews have found no technique to be superior, recommending consideration of gap length and donor site morbidity when selecting a reconstruction technique.[3,7] Younger age and increased length of follow-up were associated with improved sensory recovery.[3,7,27] Younger patients have improved axonal regeneration and greater adaptability. Improved

Table 3				
Appropriate donor nerve graft sites by anatomic zone: cross-sectional area and fascicle number				
	Zone 1	**Zone 2**	**Zone 3**	**Zone 4**
Cross-sectional area	AIN[a] PIN[a] MABCN[a]	LABCN[a]	LABCN[a]	Sural nerve
Number of fascicles	**LABCN**[a]	LABCN	**LABCN**[a]	Sural nerve

[a] Bold lettering signifies statistical significance.

Reproduced from Higgins JP, Fisher S, Serletti JM, Orlando GS. Assessment of nerve graft donor sites used for reconstruction of traumatic digital nerve defects. J Hand Surg Am. 2002;27(2):286-292. https://doi.org/10.1053/jhsu.2002

functional reorganization is seen with longer follow-up, contributing to improved outcomes.[7]

Weber and colleagues found no significant difference in outcomes between PGA conduits and nerve grafts in a randomized controlled trial. They did note that in longer gaps ($\geq$8 mm), conduits did have better outcomes than autograft. Worse 2-point discrimination was found with crush and avulsion injuries and with increasing gap size. There were 3 conduit extrusions reported.[18] Similarly, Manoli and colleagues found no significant difference between muscle-in-vein conduits and autograft, with autograft having increased donor site morbidity.[28]

In a systemic review looking at prognostic factors, reconstructions done within 15 days of injury had significantly better static 2-point discrimination than delayed reconstruction.[6] Short-segment gaps ($<$13 mm) also were found to have significantly better static 2-point discrimination.[6] Worse outcomes were observed in smokers.[6]

OTHER TECHNICAL FACTORS

Fibrin glue has been developed as an alternative to suture repair. When mixed, fibrin glue proceeds through the final pathway of blood coagulation to create a viscous adhesive that helps hold nerve ends in close approximation.[29] A randomized controlled trial comparing autologous fibrin glue with suture repair (8-0 and 9-0 epineurial repair) of median and/or ulnar nerve lacerations showed similar sensory and motor recovery, similar clinical outcomes, and similar complication rates. However, fibrin glue was found to result in a shorter operative time (6.8 min vs 22 min).[29] Two to three 8-0 or 9-0 sutures often are used when performing epineurial digital nerve suture repair.[10]

Multiple studies have investigated whether repairs done under loupe or microscope magnification affect patient outcomes. One study found no difference in sensory recovery or clinical outcomes in digital nerve repairs done under loupe magnification or the operating microscope.[30] Likewise, additional studies have found no difference when assessing median or ulnar nerve repairs done under loupe magnification or the microscope.[31,32]

SUMMARY

Multiple reconstructive options exist for digital nerve gaps that may result after adequate nerve debridement of healthy nerve ends. Options include conduit repair and autograft and allograft nerve reconstruction. Multiple comparative studies exist, with results ranging from no difference in sensory outcomes to superior recovery with allograft and autograft reconstruction as compared to conduit repair. Allograft reconstruction has been shown to have similar results to autograft reconstruction.

CLINICS CARE POINTS

- Multiple comparative studies exist addressing digital nerve defects.
- Allograft reconstruction has been shown to have similar results to autograft reconstruction.
- Several studies suggest inferior outcomes with conduit repair.

DISCLOSURE

The author has nothing to disclose.

REFERENCES

1. Wang Y, Sunitha M, Chung KC. How to measure outcomes of peripheral nerve surgery. Hand Clin 2013;29(3):349–61.
2. Mauch JT, Bae A, Shubinets V, et al. A Systematic Review of Sensory Outcomes of Digital Nerve Gap Reconstruction With Autograft, Allograft, and Conduit. Ann Plast Surg 2019;82(4S Suppl 3):S247–55.
3. Paprottka FJ, Wolf P, Harder Y, et al. Sensory recovery outcome after digital nerve repair in relation to different reconstructive techniques: meta-analysis and systematic review. Plast Surg Int 2013;2013:704589.
4. Stang F, Stollwerck P, Prommersberger KJ, et al. Posterior interosseus nerve vs. medial cutaneous nerve of the forearm: differences in digital nerve reconstruction. Arch Orthop Trauma Surg 2013;133(6):875–80.
5. Rinker BD, Ingari JV, Greenberg JA, et al. Outcomes of short-gap sensory nerve injuries reconstructed with processed nerve allografts from a multicenter registry study. J Reconstr Microsurg 2015;31(5):384–90.
6. Kim JS, Bonsu NY, Leland HA, et al. A Systematic Review of Prognostic Factors for Sensory Recovery After Digital Nerve Reconstruction. Ann Plast Surg 2018;80(5S Suppl 5):S311–6.
7. Mermans JF, Franssen BB, Serroyen J, et al. Digital nerve injuries: a review of predictors of sensory recovery after microsurgical digital nerve repair. Hand (N Y) 2012;7(3):233–41.

8. Rinker B, Zoldos J, Weber RV, et al. Use of Processed Nerve Allografts to Repair Nerve Injuries Greater Than 25 mm in the Hand. Ann Plast Surg 2017;78(6S Suppl 5):S292–5.

9. Leversedge FJ, Zoldos J, Nydick J, et al. A Multicenter Matched Cohort Study of Processed Nerve Allograft and Conduit in Digital Nerve Reconstruction. J Hand Surg Am 2020;45(12):1148–56.

10. Taras JS, Amin N, Patel N, et al. Allograft reconstruction for digital nerve loss. J Hand Surg Am 2013;38(10):1965–71.

11. Schmidhammer R, Zandieh S, Hopf R, et al. Alleviated tension at the repair site enhances functional regeneration: the effect of full range of motion mobilization on the regeneration of peripheral nerves–histologic, electrophysiologic, and functional results in a rat model. J Trauma 2004;56(3):571–84.

12. Clark WL, Trumble TE, Swiontkowski MF, et al. Nerve tension and blood flow in a rat model of immediate and delayed repairs. J Hand Surg Am 1992;17(4):677–87.

13. Driscoll PJ, Glasby MA, Lawson GM. An in vivo study of peripheral nerves in continuity: biomechanical and physiological responses to elongation. J Orthop Res 2002;20(2):370–5.

14. Yi C, Dahlin LB. Impaired nerve regeneration and Schwann cell activation after repair with tension. Neuroreport 2010;21(14):958–62.

15. Taras JS, Jacoby SM, Lincoski CJ. Reconstruction of digital nerves with collagen conduits. J Hand Surg Am 2011;36(9):1441–6.

16. Means KR Jr, Rinker BD, Higgins JP, et al. A Multicenter, Prospective, Randomized, Pilot Study of Outcomes for Digital Nerve Repair in the Hand Using Hollow Conduit Compared With Processed Allograft Nerve. Hand (N Y) 2016;11(2):144–51.

17. Haug A, Bartels A, Kotas J, et al. Sensory recovery 1 year after bridging digital nerve defects with collagen tubes. J Hand Surg Am 2013;38(1):90–7.

18. Weber RA, Breidenbach WC, Brown RE, et al. A randomized prospective study of polyglycolic acid conduits for digital nerve reconstruction in humans. Plast Reconstr Surg 2000;106(5):1036–48.

19. Mackinnon SE, Dellon AL. Clinical nerve reconstruction with a bioabsorbable polyglycolic acid tube. Plast Reconstr Surg 1990;85(3):419–24.

20. Rinker B, Liau JY. A prospective randomized study comparing woven polyglycolic acid and autogenous vein conduits for reconstruction of digital nerve gaps. J Hand Surg Am 2011;36(5):775–81.

21. Bushnell BD, McWilliams AD, Whitener GB, et al. Early clinical experience with collagen nerve tubes in digital nerve repair. J Hand Surg Am 2008;33(7):1081–7.

22. Pilanci O, Ozel A, Basaran K, et al. Is there a profit to use the lateral antebrachial cutaneous nerve as a graft source in digital nerve reconstruction? Microsurgery 2014;34(5):367–71.

23. Herman ZJ, Ilyas AM. Sensory Outcomes in Digital Nerve Repair Techniques: An Updated Meta-analysis and Systematic Review. Hand (N Y) 2020; 15(2):157–64.

24. Higgins JP, Fisher S, Serletti JM, et al. Assessment of nerve graft donor sites used for reconstruction of traumatic digital nerve defects. J Hand Surg Am 2002;27(2):286–92.

25. IJpma FF, Nicolai JP, Meek MF. Sural nerve donor-site morbidity: thirty-four years of follow-up. Ann Plast Surg 2006;57(4):391–5.

26. Cho MS, Rinker BD, Weber RV, et al. Functional outcome following nerve repair in the upper extremity using processed nerve allograft. J Hand Surg Am 2012;37(11):2340–9.

27. Kallio PK. The results of secondary repair of 254 digital nerves. J Hand Surg Br 1993;18(3):327–30.

28. Manoli T, Schulz L, Stahl S, et al. Evaluation of sensory recovery after reconstruction of digital nerves of the hand using muscle-in-vein conduits in comparison to nerve suture or nerve autografting. Microsurgery 2014;34(8):608–15.

29. Sallam A, Eldeeb M, Kamel N. Autologous Fibrin Glue Versus Microsuture in the Surgical Reconstruction of Peripheral Nerves: A Randomized Clinical Trial [published online ahead of print, 2021 May 16]. J Hand Surg Am 2021. https://doi.org/10.1016/j.jhsa.2021.03.022. S0363-5023(21)00198-2.

30. Thomas PR, Saunders RJ, Means KR. Comparison of digital nerve sensory recovery after repair using loupe or operating microscope magnification. J Hand Surg Eur Vol 2015;40(6):608–13.

31. Marsh D, Barton N. Does the use of the operating microscope improve the results of peripheral nerve suture? J Bone Joint Surg Br 1987;69(4):625–30.

32. McManamny DS. Comparison of microscope and loupe magnification: assistance for the repair of median and ulnar nerves. Br J Plast Surg 1983; 36(3):367–72.

Acute Carpal Tunnel Syndrome and Median Nerve Neurapraxia: A Review

Hayden S. Holbrook, MD, Richard A. Hillesheim, MD,
William J. Weller, MD*

KEYWORDS

• Acute carpal tunnel syndrome • Neurapraxia • Median nerve • Wrist injury • Forearm trauma

KEY POINTS

- Acute carpal tunnel syndrome after traumatic injury to the wrist is a surgical emergency requiring decompression.
- Distinguishing between acute carpal tunnel syndrome and less severe forms of median nerve neurapraxia after trauma is paramount to avoid permanent median nerve dysfunction.
- Hallmark symptoms of progressively worsening pain, and sensory disturbances in the median nerve distribution are helpful in making the diagnosis and properly treating the patient with emergent surgical release of the carpal tunnel.

INTRODUCTION

Evaluation of an acute injury to the median nerve at the wrist after trauma requires diligence, clinical acumen, and honed physical examination skills. Neuropathy after wrist trauma is a feared adverse event. It has been cited as the most common complication in some series after distal radial fractures.[1] In 1933, Abbott and Saunders first classified median neuropathy after wrist trauma into 4 clinical groups: primary injuries occurring at the time of the trauma, injuries secondary to an unreduced fragment or callus formation, injuries with late onset, and neuropathies associated with prolonged immobilization in palmar flexion (ie, the Cotton–Loder position).[2] This article will focus primarily on the first 2 etiologies mentioned insofar as they relate to acute trauma of the wrist.

Acute carpal tunnel syndrome (ACTS) and median nerve neurapraxia (MNN) both present with symptoms of median nerve dysfunction, yet their treatments differ substantially. Furthermore, failing to distinguish between the two entities can have permanent and devastating consequences for the patient. ACTS refers to a median nerve neuropathy that is *progressive* in nature, resulting from increasing pressure inside the confined space of the carpal tunnel. This diagnosis is one of the few true surgical emergencies in orthopedics and requires emergent and complete decompression of the carpal tunnel. MNN is a contusive stretch injury that occurs at the time of trauma, demonstrates nonprogressive symptoms, and is managed with expectant observation or occasionally release at the time of fracture fixation at the discretion of the surgeon. Although differentiating ACTS from MNN can be a clinical challenge, an informed clinical suspicion, focused history, and serial physical examinations can help distinguish between the two (Table 1).

ANATOMY

The carpal tunnel is an enclosed space bound by carpal bones on 3 sides and the transverse carpal ligament volary (Fig. 1). This area has a

Department of Orthopaedic Surgery and Biomedical Engineering, University of Tennessee-Campbell Clinic, Memphis, TN, USA
* Corresponding author. 1211 Union Avenue, Suite 500, Memphis, TN 38104.
E-mail address: wjweller@campbellclinic.com

Orthop Clin N Am 53 (2022) 197–203
https://doi.org/10.1016/j.ocl.2021.11.005
0030-5898/22/© 2021 Elsevier Inc. All rights reserved.

Table 1 Differentiating median nerve neurapraxia and acute carpal tunnel syndrome		
	Median Nerve Neuropraxia	**Acute Carpal Tunnel Syndrome**
Etiology	Most commonly traumatic	Numerous; trauma most common
History	Static median nerve paresthesias/dysesthesias from the time of injury	Progressive median nerve paresthesias/dysesthesias, increasing pain
Physical Examination	Static diminished 2-point discrimination	Progressive worsening 2-point discrimination, worsening Semmes-Weinstein monofilament threshold
Carpal Tunnel Pressure	Normal	Elevated
Treatment	Observation	Emergent carpal tunnel release

volume of 5 mL and a cross-sectional area of approximately 185 mm^2.[2,3] Although labeled as a tunnel and appearing to be an open compartment anatomically, the carpal tunnel functions physiologically as a closed compartment.[4] The rigid borders of the carpal tunnel leads to a rapid increase in pressure with any increase in volume. The median nerve is the only neural structure to pass through the carpal tunnel along with 9 tendons: 4 superficialis tendons, 4 profundus tendons, and the flexor pollicis longus (FPL) tendon. On exiting the carpal tunnel, the median nerve supplies sensation to the radial 3.5 digits and motor innervation to the thenar musculature, as well as the lumbricals of the index and long fingers. The palmar cutaneous branch of the median nerve arises proximal to the carpal tunnel and supplies sensation to the radial aspect of the palm. This area is spared with compression of the median nerve at the carpal tunnel.

ACUTE CARPAL TUNNEL SYNDROME

The etiologies of ACTS are extensive, but they all share an acute increase in carpal tunnel pressure as the central mechanism of injury. ACTS most commonly occurs after traumatic injuries to the wrist, including distal radial fractures, perilunate or lunate dislocations, carpal and metacarpal fractures, among others.[5] Traumatic ACTS usually results from hemorrhage into the carpal tunnel, fracture edema, or reduction in carpal tunnel volume from impinging fracture fragments. Numerous case reports have been presented on atraumatic causes of ACTS (infectious, inflammatory, coagulopathic, anatomic, fluid imbalance, and oncologic origins) but these are rare in comparison to traumatic causes.[5] A

key to understanding the seriousness of an ACTS diagnosis is that it is akin to acute compartment syndrome of the leg, thigh, or forearm. That is to say, the increase in tunnel pressure threatens perfusion to the median nerve as the pressure equalizes between the carpal tunnel and the incoming capillary blood flow. Similarly, obstruction of venous outflow can lead to endoneurial edema, rising endoneurial pressure, and ultimately a "mini" compartment syndrome within the fascicle when the perineurium is intact.[6,7] Endoneurial edema also interrupts axonal conduction through altered axonal ionic environment. Lundborg and colleagues provided evidence using a human model that ischemia is the driving force of neuropathy, not mechanical compression alone.[8] In addition, a dose-responsive reaction to an induced carpal tunnel syndrome has been demonstrated in a rabbit model.[9] As compartmental pressures increased, a shorter time was required to induce a complete conduction block. Carpal tunnel pressures within 30 mm Hg of diastolic blood pressure can cause median nerve motor and sensory dysfunction.[10,11] Thus, hypertensive patients with elevated perfusion pressures may better tolerate increased carpal tunnel pressure. The opposite is true for a hypotensive patient or one in shock.[10]

MEDIAN NERVE NEURAPRAXIA

MNN describes the first group classified by Abbott and Saunders (primary injury occurring at the time of trauma).[1] MNN is typically a nerve injury that results from a variety of mechanisms in combination or in isolation. These include tenting or stretching of the nerve over a fractured or dislocated bone fragment, or direct

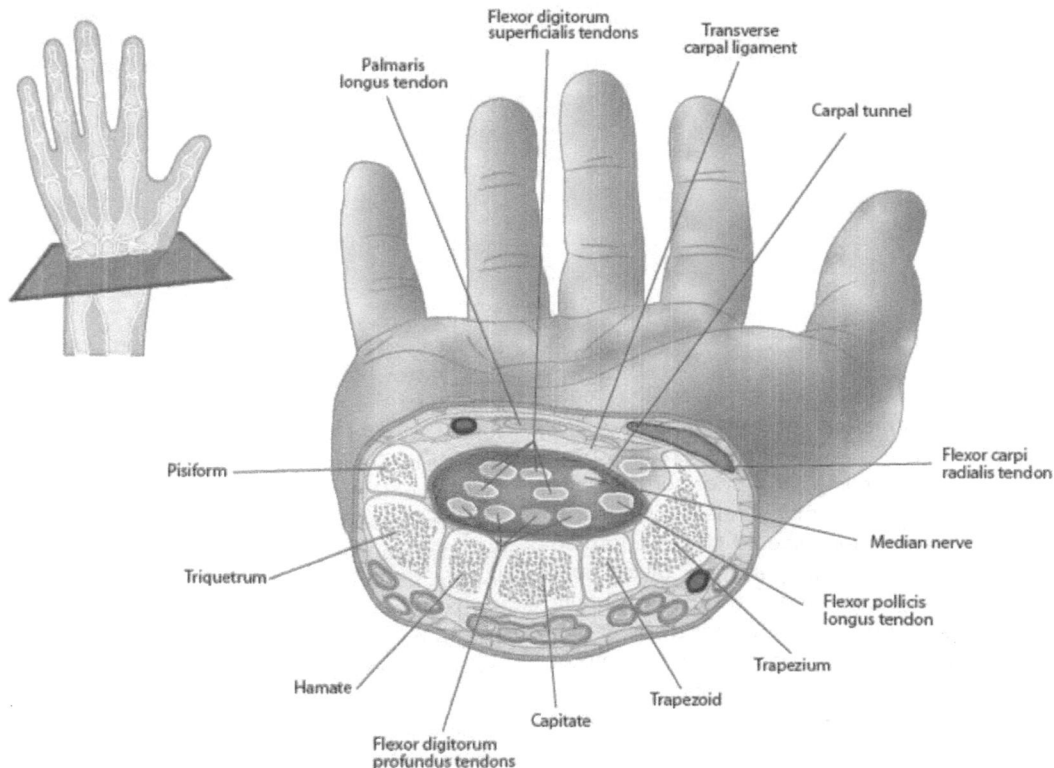

Fig. 1. Anatomy of the carpal tunnel.

neurapraxia of the nerve by an internal or external force (Fig. 2).[12] Neurapraxia occurs with maximal deformity of the wrist at the time of the injury, and thus patients present with immediate and nonprogressive median nerve dysfunction. Neurotmesis of the median nerve has been reported in the setting of high-energy distal radial fractures.[13]

DIAGNOSIS

The differential diagnosis of a median neuropathy after wrist trauma includes MNN, ACTS, forearm compartment syndrome, and exacerbation of a chronic underlying carpal tunnel syndrome.[14] Differentiating between these 4 entities is critical but possible through a detailed history and physical examination. The primary focus of this article will be on MNN and ACTS.

HISTORY

After primary evaluation according to Advanced Trauma Life Support guidelines is complete, a detailed history should be obtained from the patient or, if necessary, next of kin. The mechanism of injury should be investigated to understand the level of energy imparted to the wrist

structures. A medical and surgical history should be obtained, and the presence of any preceding symptoms of median or peripheral neuropathy should be elicited. Current medications, specifically blood thinners, may predispose the patient to the development of a compressive hematoma and should be discussed with him or her. Finally, the patient should be evaluated for the presence or absence of paresthesias or dysesthesias. When present, the discerning physician must determine (1) the onset of these subjective sensations (at the time of the injury, delayed, or longstanding deficits BEFORE the* injury) and (2) whether these symptoms are progressively worsening or remaining stable. Patients who develop ACTS present with median nerve symptoms that start after the injury and worsen within a relatively short period of hours. On initial presentation patients may report a normal sensory examination, and it is not until later that sensory changes and worsening pain develop as edema increases.[15] In contrast, MNN sensory deficits remain static from the time of the injury and may improve after reduction and with time. Pain also improves in MNN after reduction, whereas ACTS has progressive deficits and worsening pain.

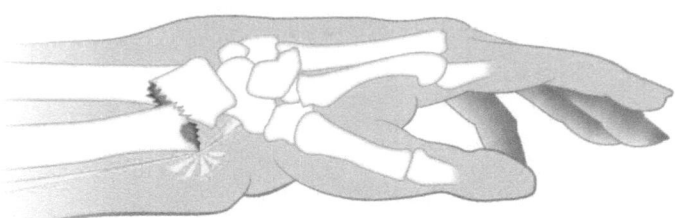

Fig. 2. Bony displacement at the time of injury may result in a neurapraxic injury to the median nerve.

PHYSICAL EXAMINATION

The physical examination provides the most important information in distinguishing ACTS from MNN. The skin should be examined for open wounds, swelling, and prior surgical incisions such as a carpal tunnel release incision. A vascular examination should be performed ensuring adequate distal perfusion, taking note of capillary refill time, and, if necessary, obtaining radial and ulnar digital artery Doppler signals. A detailed sensory and motor examination will be most diagnostic.

Sensation can be assessed with static 2-point discrimination, moving/dynamic 2-point discrimination, Semmes–Weinstein monofilament tests, and vibration sense.[11] Static discrimination and moving/dynamic 2-point discrimination test innervation density as multiple overlapping sensory inputs along with intact cortical integration are required. A normal static 2-point discrimination is less than 6 mm and less than 3 mm when assessed dynamically (Fig. 3).[16] Because 2-point discrimination may remain intact with only a few conducting nerve fibers, these are not as sensitive to a gradual decline in nerve function seen during neural compression such as in ACTS. Semmes-Weinstein monofilament and vibration tests are examples of a threshold test measuring input from a single nerve fiber and its associated receptors. An experimental model of ACTS has shown that abnormalities in Semmes-Weinstein monofilament are detected significantly earlier than changes in 2-point discrimination.[10] These findings suggest that waiting for a change in 2-point discrimination may delay the diagnosis and treatment of ACTS. However, we recommend performing and documenting sensibility testing with both 2-point discrimination and, if available, Semmes–Weinstein monofilament from the onset.

Motor assessment of the median nerve also should be performed, though in the traumatic setting this can be limited because of a patient's lack of cooperation secondary to pain. On repeated examination in ACTS, worsening motor function may be appreciated. The recurrent motor branch, which is the terminal motor branch of the median nerve distal to the carpal tunnel, should be assessed with palmar abduction of the thumb via the abductor pollicis brevis. Documenting motor function of the median nerve by assessing flexion strength of the thumb interphalangeal joint through the flexor pollicis longus (FPL) is incorrect and misleading in this setting because the FPL is innervated proximal to the carpal tunnel through the anterior interosseous nerve (AIN). Note, often motor assessment in the context of trauma is difficult due to patient guarding, anxiety, pain, and bony instability, thus deficiencies in motor function strength will likely be noted and should be documented accordingly. Serial evaluation of subjective dysesthesias with objective motor and sensory examinations is the most vital aspect in diagnosing ACTS.

In comparison, patients with MNN will present with diminished or absent sensation in the median nerve distribution of the hand from the onset. This should be assessed in the same manner as described above as well as a motor examination. Symptoms of MNN are static sensory abnormalities seen immediately at the time of injury and typically do not progress and often improve after reduction or immobilization. Additionally, pain often is much improved after reduction in patients with MNN.

COMPARTMENT PRESSURE MONITORING

Carpal tunnel compartment pressure serves as another objective tool for evaluation and diagnosis of ACTS and to differentiate it from MNN. Multiple techniques have been reported for placement of a catheter probe within the carpal tunnel to obtain a pressure reading. Commercial devices are available such as the intracompartmental pressure monitor system (Stryker, Kalamazoo, MI). The catheter needle is inserted 1 cm proximal to the distal wrist crease just ulnar to the palmaris longus or in line with the ring finger. The needle is positioned

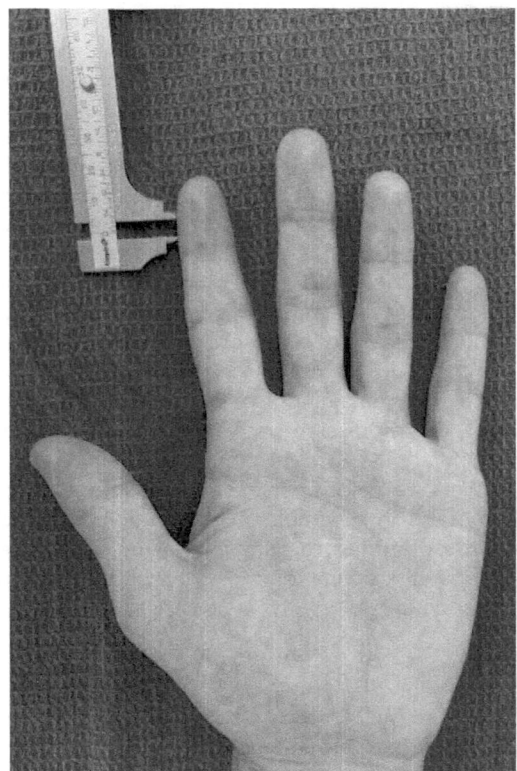

Fig. 3. Two-point discrimination testing is a critical part of the physical examination when assessing for MNN and median nerve contusion.

at a 45-degree angle, aimed slightly radially, and advanced until the needle reaches the floor of the carpal tunnel. The needle is retracted a millimeter to prevent tissues from blocking the needle tip.

In a normal hand, the pressure within the carpal tunnel is approximately 2.5 mm Hg, but this pressure increases with wrist flexion and extension.[17] In a human model of ACTS, Gelberman and colleagues reported that a critical block in motor and sensory function occurs between 40 and 50 mm Hg, with some functional loss occurring at 40 mm Hg and complete loss at 50 mm Hg.[18,19] From their work, they recommended the release of the carpal tunnel if pressures exceed 40 mm Hg. Dresing and colleagues measured carpal tunnel pressures in 56 patients with distal radial fractures that averaged 23 mm Hg on presentation.[20] They also showed that carpal tunnel pressure correlated with the severity of the fracture pattern. Mack and colleagues reported an elevated average carpal tunnel pressure of 52 mm Hg (range, 40–60 mm Hg) in 4 of 5 patients with ACTS after wrist trauma. The fifth patient with a normal

pressure recording was noted to have a misplaced catheter at the time of surgery. They also reported carpal tunnel pressures of 5 and 6 mm Hg at 5 and 13 days in 2 patients with MNN.[21] Although objective measurement of the carpal tunnel compartment pressure can help differentiate ACTS from MNN, the accuracy and reliability of a detailed history and physical examination limit the application of this invasive diagnostic tool.

IMAGING

Radiographs should be obtained in the setting of trauma. Advanced imaging is rarely indicated in the setting of ACTS and will only delay treatment but may be beneficial for preoperative planning when simultaneous fracture fixation is planned at the time of carpal tunnel release. The physician should recognize injury patterns that predispose to ACTS and heighten their clinical suspicion for the development of this complication. For example, Dyer and colleagues showed that operatively treated distal radial fractures with translation greater than 35% and women less than 48 years of age were the most highly correlated with the development of ACTS.[22] ACTS has been reported to complicate 23% to 45% of perilunate dislocations.[23,24] When a high-risk injury pattern is recognized, a 2-point discrimination measurement should be obtained and documented at the first encounter and serial examinations performed every 4 hours.

TREATMENT

Once the diagnosis of ACTS has been made, treatment is emergent carpal tunnel release. Because ACTS is most commonly related to traumatic injuries to the forearm, wrist, and hand, careful preoperative incision planning is necessary. Decompression in the setting of ACTS requires a more extensile incision for full evaluation of the traumatized soft tissues compared to that of an elective release of chronic carpal tunnel syndrome. As with a standard carpal tunnel release, one should avoid injury to the motor recurrent branch of the median nerve, superficial palmar arch distally, and ensure complete release of the entire transverse carpal ligament and distal forearm fascia. Hematoma within the carpal tunnel, the common culprit for ACTS, should be evacuated.

For ACTS associated with a distal radial fracture, a 2-incision technique should be performed when volar plating is performed simultaneously.

Although a single incision can be used through a flexor carpi radialis (FCR) approach that continues into a carpal tunnel incision, this risks injury to the palmar cutaneous branch of the median nerve residing in the ulnar aspect of the FCR tendon sheath.[25,26] The 2-incision approach uses a longitudinal palmar incision for carpal tunnel release and a volar Henry approach or trans-FCR approach instead. The extended FCR approach has been shown to be safe and effective for treatment of distal radial fractures when compared with a classic volar Henry approach.[27]

Management and outcomes after MNN is defined by the degree of median nerve injury: neurapraxia, axonotmesis, or neurotmesis.[13,28] Neurapraxia is the most common type of injury, and observation is typically all that is required, although release at the time of fracture fixation is at the surgeon's discretion.[14] If the median nerve continues to be stretched by a displaced bone fragment, a closed reduction should be urgently performed.[12] The fracture can be definitively treated at a later time if the median nerve symptoms improve after reduction. The neurapraxia is expected to gradually improve with time.

TIMING AND OUTCOMES

Early differentiation between ACTS and MNN ensures timely treatment and improved outcomes. As urgent decompression of the carpal tunnel is recommended upon diagnosis of ACTS, delay in diagnosis or treatment may result in poor recovery. Patients with ACTS treated with early carpal tunnel release have earlier and more complete resolution of median nerve dysfunction.[15,21,29] Mack and colleagues have reported a series of 10 patients with ACTS after wrist trauma. Eight patients were treated with carpal tunnel release between 4 hours and 33 days after onset of sensory deficits, and the other 2 were managed with elevation, cast splitting, and observation. Of the 4 patients treated early between 4 and 40 hours, all reported normal sensation by 96 hours after decompression. A fifth patient treated early at 20 hours reported subjective numbness but had a normal 2-point discrimination examination at 3 months. Three patients were treated in a delayed fashion at 6, 9, and 33 days, and each had persistent median nerve dysesthesias at 3 months.[21] Ford and Ali reported 5 patients with ACTS after wrist trauma. Four patients underwent carpal tunnel release at 14 hours, 36 hours, 72 hours, and 1 week after injury and each reported residual median nerve symptoms that persisted at

10 months, resolved at 4 months, persisted at 4 months, and persisted at 6 months, respectively. One patient underwent decompression of the carpal tunnel within 3 hours of injury and had no signs of median nerve dysfunction 12 hours postoperatively.[15] Bauman and colleagues reported ACTS in 5 patients following immobilization in wrist flexion for wrist trauma who were initially treated with cast splitting and repositioning. Patients were monitored for improvement of symptoms before proceeding with surgical decompression. One patient improved with only conservative measures alone. The remaining 4 patients underwent surgical decompression between 36 and 96 hours after injury. At 8 to 14-month follow-up, 3 of 4 patients revealed persistent dysesthesias and numbness in the median distribution.[29] Based on these studies, urgent carpal tunnel release is generally recommended within 8 hours of an ACTS diagnosis.

SUMMARY

ACTS and MNN often present similarly in the immediate posttraumatic period but can be differentiated through a focused history and serial physical examinations. The time course of ACTS may be variable but is defined by progressively worsening pain and sensory changes in the median nerve distribution. This is secondary to increasing compartmental pressure within the tunnel, which could eventually equalize incoming capillary perfusion or even obstruct venous outflow. Irreparable and devastating median nerve damage can occur under these conditions, and emergent carpal tunnel release is indicated.

CLINICS CARE POINTS

- Acute carpal tunnel syndrome is a true surgical emergency. Progressively worsening pain and sensory changes are hallmark signs of acute carpal tunnel syndrome.

- Failing to distinguish acute carpal tunnel from median nerve neurapraxia can have permanent devastating consequences. Physical examination and compartment pressure measurements provide the most important information in making the diagnosis.

- Once acute carpal tunnel syndrome is determined, emergent carpal tunnel release is required.

FINANCIAL DISCLOSURE

The authors have no financial disclosures and report no conflicts of interest.

REFERENCES

1. Cooney WP 3rd, Dobyns JH, Lindscheid RL. Complications of Colles' fractures. J Bone Joint Surg Am 1980;62(4):613–9.
2. Abbott LC, Saunders JB. Injuries of median nerve in fractures of lower end of radius. Surg Gynecol Obstet 1933;57(Oct):507–16.
3. Rotman MB, Donovan JP. Practical anatomy of the carpal tunnel. Hand Clin 2002;18(2):219–30.
4. Cobb TK, Cooney WP, An KN. Pressure dynamics of the carpal tunnel and flexor compartment of the forearm. J Hand Surg Am 1995;20(2):193–8.
5. Gillig JD, White SD, Rachel JN. Acute carpal tunnel syndrome: a review of current literature. Orthop Clin North Am 2016;47(3):599–607.
6. Lundborg G, Myers R, Powell H. Nerve compression injury and increased endoneurial fluid pressure a "miniature compartment syndrome. J Neurol Neurosurg Psychiatry 1983;46(12):1119–24.
7. Schnetzler KA. Acute carpal tunnel syndrome. J Am Acad Orthop Surg 2008;16(5):276–82.
8. Lundborg G, Gelberman RH, Minteer-Convery M, et al. Median nerve compression in the carpal tunnel-functional response to experimentally induced controlled pressure. J Hand Surg Am 1982;7(3):252–9.
9. Lim JY, Cho SH, Han TR, et al. Dose-responsiveness of electrophysiologic change in a new model of acute carpal tunnel syndrome. Clin Orthop Relat Res 2004;427:120–6.
10. Szabo RM, Gelberman RH. Peripheral nerve compression: etiology, critical pressure threshold, and clinical assessment. Orthopedics 1984;7(9):1461–6.
11. Szabo RM. Acute carpal tunnel syndrome. Hand Clin 1998;14(3):419–29.
12. Waters PM, Kolettis GJ, Schwend R. Acute median neuropathy following physeal fractures of the distal radius. J Pediatr Orthop 1994;14(2):173–7.
13. Swan CC, Buchanan PJ, Chim H. Complete transection of the median nerve with distal radius fracture: a case report. JBJS Case Connect 2020;10(2):e0328.
14. Floyd WE 4th, Earp BE, Blazar PE. Acute median nerve problems in the setting of a distal radius fracture. J Hand Surg Am 2015;40(8):1669–71.
15. Ford DJ, Ali MS. Acute carpal tunnel syndrome. Complications of delayed decompression. J Bone Joint Surg Br 1986;68(5):758–9.
16. Kenney RJ, Hammert WC. Physical examination of the hand. J Hand Surg Am 2014;39(11):2324–34.
17. Gelberman RH, Hergenroeder PT, Hargens AR, et al. The carpal tunnel syndrome. A study of carpal canal pressures. J Bone Joint Surg Am 1981;63(3):380–3.
18. Gelberman RH, Szabo RM, Williamson RV, et al. Sensibility testing in peripheral-nerve compression syndromes. An experimental study in humans. J Bone Joint Surg Am 1983;65(5):632–8.
19. Gelberman RH, Szabo RM, Williamson RV, et al. Tissue pressure threshold for peripheral nerve viability. Clin Orthop Relat Res 1983;178:285–91.
20. Dresing K, Peterson T, Schmit-Neuerburg KP. Compartment pressure in the carpal tunnel in distal fractures of the radius. A prospective study. Arch Orthop Trauma Surg 1994;113(5):286–9.
21. Mack GR, McPherson SA, Lutz RB. Acute median neuropathy after wrist trauma. The role of emergent carpal tunnel release. Clin Orthop Relat Res 1994;300:141–6.
22. Dyer G, Lozano-Calderon S, Gannon C, et al. Predictors of acute carpal tunnel syndrome associated with fracture of the distal radius. J Hand Surg Am 2008;33(8):1309–13.
23. Sotereanos DG, Mitsionis GJ, Giannakopoulos PN, et al. Perilunate dislocation and fracture dislocation: a critical analysis of the volar-dorsal approach. J Hand Surg Am 1997;22(1):49–56.
24. Knoll VD, Allan C, Trumble TE. Trans-scaphoid perilunate fracture dislocations: results of screw fixation of the scaphoid and lunotriquetral repair with a dorsal approach. J Hand Surg Am 2005;30(6):1145–52.
25. Pensy RA, Brunton LM, Parks BG, et al. Single-incision extensile volar approach to the distal radius and concurrent carpal tunnel release: cadaveric study. J Hand Surg Am 2010;35(2):217–22.
26. Avis D, Power D. Letter regarding "The extended flexor carpi radialis approach for concurrent carpal tunnel release and volar plate osteosynthesis for distal radius fracture. J Hand Surg Am 2016;41(5):e111.
27. Tannan SC, Pappou IP, Gwathmey FW, et al. The extended flexor carpi radialis approach for concurrent carpal tunnel release and volar plate osteosynthesis for distal radius fracture. J Hand Surg Am 2015;40(10):2026–31.
28. Dennison DG. Median nerve injuries associated with distal radius fractures. Tech Orthop 2006;21(1):48–53.
29. Bauman TD, Gelberman RH, Mubarak SJ, et al. The acute carpal tunnel syndrome. Clin Orthop Relat Res 1981;156:151–6.

Shoulder and Elbow

Incidence, Risk Factors, Prevention, and Management of Peripheral Nerve Injuries Following Shoulder Arthroplasty

Manan S. Patel, MD[a], Mohammad Daher, BSc[b],
David A. Fuller, MD[c], Joseph A. Abboud, MD[d],*

KEYWORDS

- Reverse total shoulder arthroplasty • Anatomic total shoulder arthroplasty • Neuromonitoring
- Nerve injury • Prevention • Management

KEY POINTS

- Iatrogenic nerve injuries following shoulder arthroplasty are cited at 1% to 18.7% in the current literature, whereas distal peripheral neuropathies occur in 1% to 12.3% of patients.
- Thorough physical examination is required in the postoperative period to screen for neurologic injuries, given that symptomology is masked by postoperative pain and functional restriction.
- Causes of nerve injury include direct and indirect causes. Direct causes include laceration and compression from retractor use and indirect causes include arm positioning and lengthening
- Neurologic deficits should be worked-up with electrodiagnostic studies no earlier than 3-week following surgery and can be performed serially to look for signs of reinnervation, as most iatrogenic nerve injuries resolve in 6 to 12 months.
- For high-grade, neurotmesis type injuries, primary end-to-end, neurorrhaphy or nerve reconstruction with a tension-free graft should be performed as soon as possible, whereas patients who have persistent evidence of nerve injury should be considered for exploration with treatment via neurolysis, nerve grafts, nerve transfers, or muscle/tendon transfers.

INTRODUCTION

Anatomic (aTSA) and reverse total shoulder arthroplasty (rTSA) utilization is increasing at rates faster than those of total hip and total knee arthroplasties, with increases in use of 103.7% and 191.3% from 2011 to 2017, respectively.[1] As the prevalence of patients living with primary shoulder replacements surges, so does the number of patients who may require revision surgery.[2] Given this, complications that affect patient function, such as infection, hematoma, component loosening, scapular notching, nerve injury, and continued postoperative pain and stiffness, can lead to morbidity and significant burden on health care systems.[2–4]

Iatrogenic neurologic injury following TSA is cited at an incidence of 1% to 18.7%.[5–10] Most of these injuries are thought to result from inadvertent traction of the brachial plexus during

---

[a] Department of Orthopaedic Surgery, Cooper University Hospital, Camden, NJ, USA; [b] Faculty of Medicine, Saint-Joseph University, Beirut, Lebanon; [c] Department of Orthopaedic Surgery, Cooper Medical School of Rowan University, Camden, NJ, USA; [d] Department of Orthopaedic Surgery, The Rothman Institute at Thomas Jefferson University, Rothman Orthopaedic Institute at Thomas Jefferson University, 925 Chestnut Street 5th Floor, Philadelphia, PA 19107, USA
* Corresponding author:
E-mail address: abboudj@gmail.com

Orthop Clin N Am 53 (2022) 205–213
https://doi.org/10.1016/j.ocl.2021.11.006
0030-5898/22/© 2021 Elsevier Inc. All rights reserved.

retraction, particularly in the extremes of shoulder range of motion.[11–13] Other sources of potential injury include direct laceration during dissection, trauma from interscalene block anesthesia, pull on plexus from lengthened limb, and vascular injury and/or compression from hematoma or retractor use.[4–7,11,14–16] Reported injuries vary from neuropraxia to neurotmesis, resulting in a spectrum of symptomology from transitory pain to devastating loss of upper extremity function.[6,16] Moreover, although not well understood, there is a reported incidence of new-onset distal peripheral neuropathy (DPN) of the median, ulnar, and radial nerves following aTSA and rTSA of 7.1% and 12.3%, respectively.[17]

The purpose of this review is to characterize nerve injuries following primary and revision shoulder arthroplasty, including incidence, risk factors, and methods of prevention.

INCIDENCE

The incidence of neurologic complications after TSA is challenging to estimate due to the fact that clinical presentation may be subclinical in the early postoperative period.[14] The factors contributing to this underestimation are the limited neurologic examination due to the postoperative pain and functional restriction—some nerve dysfunction may be transient and resolve before proper clinical examination.[14] In fact, studies that made use of electromyography (EMG) to diagnose nerve injury following TSA, postoperatively, have reported much higher incidences of 16% to 22%.[5,16] In studies not making use of EMG in the postoperative period, neurologic symptomology in patients undergoing TSA is cited at 1% to 18.7%.[5–10]

A thorough clinical examination is necessary to properly elucidate neurologic dysfunction in the postoperative period. Ball and colleagues examined 211 TSA patients. He reported 44 postoperative neurologic complications in 211 patients after TSA (20.9%); however, only 38 were directly related to the surgery (18%). All but 4 of these patients had symptom resolution by 1 year, and all were symptom free by 2 years.[14] The rate of nerve injury in his patient population is on the higher end of the spectrum, likely due to his thorough physical examination to screen for this specific dysfunction.

Patients may also develop DPN following TSA at rates of 1.9% to 12.3%.[14,17,18] In the Ball and colleagues study, of the 6 patients who he defined as sustaining neurologic injury not related to the surgery, 2 had cervical pathology

and 4 (1.9%) developed DPN (2 carpel tunnel, 2 ulnar neuropathy).[14] Yian and colleagues evaluated 606 shoulder replacements (319 aTSA, 168 hemiarthroplasties, 71 rTSA, 31 humeral resurfacing, and 17 revision TSA) and found a DPN rate of 2.5% (10 carpel tunnel, 5 cubital tunnel).[18] Thomasson and colleagues reported DPN in 6 (7.1%) patients undergoing aTSA and in 7 (12.3%) patients undergoing rTSA; these included cubital tunnel, carpal tunnel, and 2 radial sensory neuropathies.[17]

CAUSES AND RISK FACTORS

Nerve injury in shoulder arthroplasty can be direct[14,19,20] or indirect[5,14,16,19] such as laceration during surgical dissection or compression secondary to retractor use versus excessive traction from shoulder positioning or arm lengthening from hardware implantation or compressive pressure from postoperative hematoma formation, respectively. Other general causes include operative time, surgeon experience, and revision surgery.[5,19,21–24] In addition, although the mechanism is not entirely elucidated, postoperative swelling and immobilization can lead to DPNs.[17]

Indirect Causes

Inadvertent traction on the brachial plexus applied intraoperatively during different arm positions can cause nerve stress and is thought to be one of the main causes of injury. Lenoir and colleagues performed a cadaveric study in 10 shoulders evaluating nerve tension on the brachial plexus during the course of a rTSA procedure. Before any implantation of hardware, the investigators found that internal rotation (IR) increased stress on the radial and axillary nerves, whereas external rotation (ER) stressed the musculocutaneous, median, and ulnar nerves; extension placed stress on all of the nerves. During the course of rTSA surgery, humeral exposure, particularly when the arm was placed in extension, and glenoid exposure placed the largest stress on nerves.[25] In another cadaveric study, performed by Kam and colleagues on 6 cadavers undergoing hemiarthroplasty or revision rTSA, evaluated combinations of arm range of motion that applied greater than 10% strain on the plexus, which they defined as adequate strain to cause nerve injury based on animal studies. They found that combined shoulder abduction greater than 70°, ER greater than 60°, and extension of greater than 50° increased medial cord tension to greater than the threshold. In addition, when the elbow was supported, all specimens experienced less stress.[26]

Arm lengthening during rTSA is a known cause of nerve injury due to indirect pull on the brachial plexus. Lädermann and colleagues evaluated patients for neurologic injury following aTSA and rTSA via EMG in the postoperative period. In the rTSA, the investigators used a *Grammont*-style rTSA system that lengthened the arm by a mean 27 mm. In patients with no prior history of upper extremity neurologic symptoms, patients with EMG positive nerve injury had their arms lengthened at a mean of 42 mm compared with those who were EMG negative at 26 mm. Given their small sample size, the investigators were unable to give a precise number for amount of lengthening that could be tolerated from neurologic standpoint.[16] That number likely lies greater than 20 mm, as shown in a recent study by Kim and colleagues, in which the they evaluated 34 (18.7%) nerve injuries in 182 consecutive rTSA. The investigators showed a significant difference in arm lengthening in those who suffered an injury compared with those who did not (postoperative acromiohumeral distance: 34.1 ± 11.0 mm vs 29.4 ± 7.6 mm [$P = .015$]; postoperative distalization: 24.5 ± 9.4 mm vs 20.5 ± 8.3 mm [$P = .009$]).[10] In addition, in a cadaveric study by Marion and colleagues, when the humerus was lowered below the equator of the glenoid there was increased stretch and tension on the axillary nerve. However, in humeri that were lateralized, as opposed to lengthened, stretching of the nerve was absent.[27]

Glenoid exposure is associated with increased stress on the axillary, musculocutaneous, and radial nerves.[25] In fact, Nagda and colleagues used intraoperative nerve monitoring (IONM) in 30 shoulders undergoing TSA and reported that 50% of the motor evoked potentials (MEPs) occurred during glenoid exposure, and 50% of MEPs occurred as well when the arm was positioned in ER, abduction, and extension.[5]

Direct Causes

Various points during the course of a case cause increased tension on the brachial plexus, such as glenoid or humeral head exposure, as mentioned by Lenoir and colleagues.[25] In this study, the investigators found that when retractors were placed between the anterior deltoid muscle and the conjoint tendon for exposition of the humerus there was a significant increase in stress on the musculocutaneous, radial, and median nerves when arm is extended greater

than 60°.[25] The musculocutaneous nerve pierces the coracobrachialis and the short head of the biceps and thus can be protected by avoiding aggressive retractor use on the conjoint tendon. Similarly, if a deltoid splitting approach is used, prolonged retractor use can cause damage to the axillary nerve that runs 5 to 7 cm from the acromial edge.[28]

During glenoid preparation for rTSA implantation, integrity of the axillary nerve may be endangered due to its proximity to the inferior glenoid rim and the humeral metaphysis, as well as when reaming the humeral metaphysis to avoid posterior humeral cortical injury.[29] Lastly, during placement of the glenoid baseplate, the suprascapular nerve may be injured due to extraosseous screw placement during both superior and posterior drilling.[29–31] The placement of the posterior screw imparts the highest risk to the nerve, whereas the inferior screw exhibits little to no risk.[32]

General Considerations

Understandably longer operations, whether that is due to difficulty of case, intraoperative complications, and/or surgeon experience, will increase the risk of complications, including neurologic ones. In a database study by Wilson and colleagues, which included 10,082 patients who underwent TSA, the investigators found that there is an 88% increased risk of peripheral nerve injuries with each 20 minutes added to the operative time.[21] Revision TSA, which is inherently more complex than primary TSA given requirement of osteotomies for implant removal, surgical dissection through scarred tissue planes, and/or reconstruction of soft tissue or any osseous defects, can also increase the risk of nerve injury.[24] Lastly, surgeon experience may play a factor in neurologic injury as well, particularly early in one's career.[22]

PREVENTION

With cautious awareness of the direct and indirect multifactorial causes of nerve injury in TSA, neurologic morbidities can be avoided in patients. The surgeon can take many steps to minimize the neurologic risks associated with shoulder arthroplasty surgery in the primary and/or revision settings.

Prevention begins with a strong understanding of the anatomic relationships of the brachial plexus nerves within the shoulder in order to avoid any direct trauma—particularly to axillary, suprascapular, and musculocutaneous nerves.[33] Important anatomic areas to be cognizant

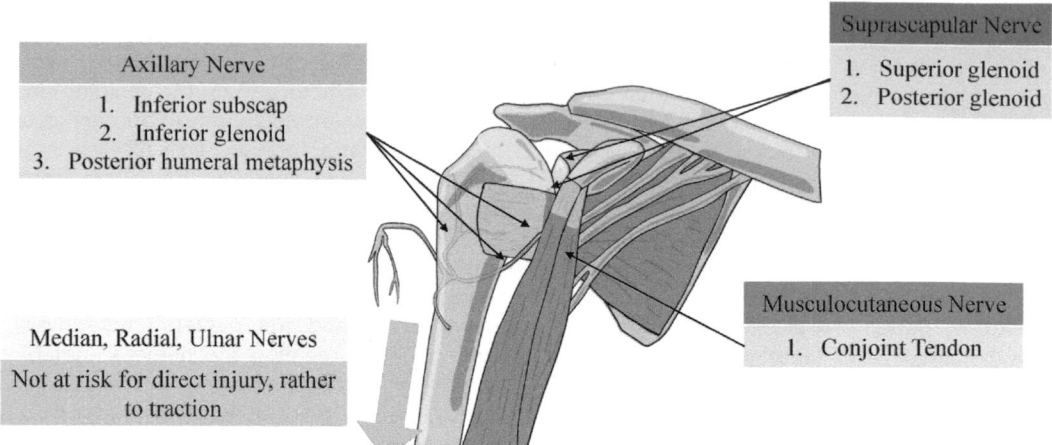

Fig. 1. Depicts the common anatomical areas of nerve injury for each of the major nerves in the shoulder that are at risk.

during the course of the case are shown in (**Fig. 1**). The axillary nerve is at increased risk of injury at 3 specific anatomic landmarks. First, it passes obliquely below the inferior border of the subscapularis into the quadrangular space, about 0 to 12 mm from the subscapularis insertion, and thus care should be taken when mobilizing the subscapularis.[34,35] Second, the nerve is vulnerable at the inferior glenoid rim between the 5:30 and 6:30 positions relative to glenoid face.[29,36–38] The literature is inconsistent on the distance of the nerve from the glenoid, particularly at different arm positions, hence, any inferior glenoid work should be undertaken under direct visualization. Lastly, the distance between the axillary nerve and the posterior humeral metaphysis ranges from 0.6 to 21.3 mm in cadaveric studies.[29,39] The suprascapular nerve is at risk from screw placement superiorly and posteriorly in the glenoid. A safe zone was developed by Shishido and Kikuchi of limiting screw length to less than 23 mm and less than 14 mm, superiorly and posteriorly, respectively, to avoid suprascapular nerve injury.[40] The musculocutaneous nerve pierces the coracobrachialis muscle at 22 to 86 mm from the inferior tip of the coracoid.[41] The nerve is at highest risk during prolonged retractor tension placed on the conjoint tendon. Radial, median, and ulnar nerves are generally not at risk for direct injury in this anatomic plane and are most susceptible to indirect traction from arm positioning and/or lengthening.

Attention must be paid to the indirect causes of nerve trauma as well. As mentioned, IR increased stress on the radial and axillary nerves, ER stresses the musculocutaneous, median, and

ulnar nerves, and extension placed stress all of the nerves.[25] In addition, combined shoulder abduction greater than 70°, ER greater than 60°, and extension of greater than 50° increase medial cord tension to greater than the threshold of 10%. Furthermore, when the elbow is supported, all nerves experience less stress.[26] Hence, minimizing the use of these specific range of motion parameters, while supporting the elbow during the course of the case, can decrease the stress placed on the plexus.

During rTSA, lengthening of the arm should be avoided, as that has been shown to increase traction on the brachial plexus. In our study, in which 191 patients who underwent rTSA, we found zero brachial plexus injuries in the postoperative period—note that 9 patients suffered DPNs. All rTSA in this study used a lateralized design that minimized lengthening.[42]

One particular intervention that can serve as a preventative measure is continuous IONM. As neurologic dysfunction during the course of shoulder surgery is dynamic, IONM provides real-time feedback to the surgeon of any impending nerve stress, thereby allowing him/her to intervene intraoperatively to avoid or minimize any true injury. In general, IONM leads are placed, subdermally, in the muscle bellies that represent each of the major 5 nerves of the upper extremity to monitor for transcranial MEP, and 2 additional electrodes are placed superficially over the ulnar and median and ulnar nerves to monitor somatosensory evoked potentials (SSEP) (**Fig. 2**); free run EMG is run as well. Both arms are prepped in this fashion, and stimulating electrodes are placed extracranially. A

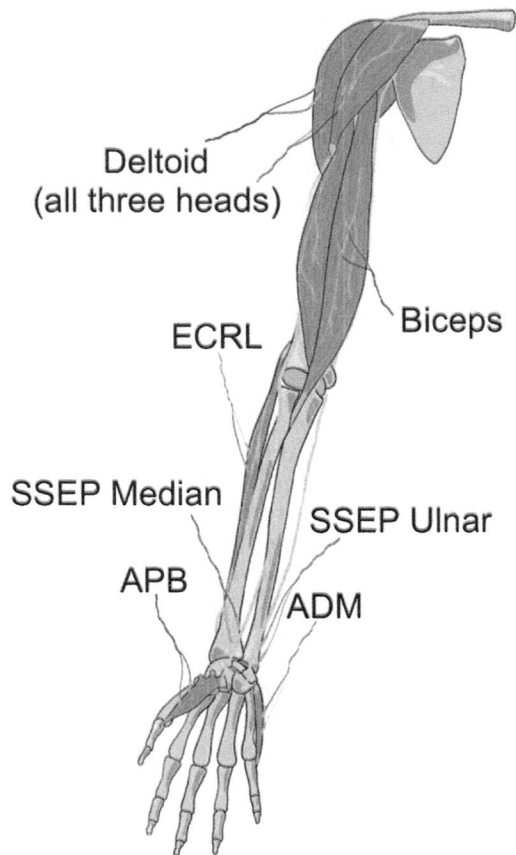

Deltoid
(all three heads)

ECRL

Biceps

SSEP Median

SSEP Ulnar

APB

ADM

Fig. 2. Depicts lead placement for intraoperative nerve monitoring. Leads are placed in the muscle belly that represent each of the five major nerves of the upper extremity. Two additional leads are placed superficially over the median and ulnar nerve to monitor sensory function (ie, SSEP median and SSEP ulnar). ADM, abductor digiti minimi; APB, abductor pollicis brevis; ECRL, extensor carpi radialis longus; SSEP2, somatosensory evoked potential.

neurophysiologist watches over the case and notifies the surgical team of any alerts.

The authors performed 2 recent IONM studies in primary[42] and revision TSA,[43] in which they reported no major or minor nerve injuries in either study with 3.1% and 9.1% DPN rate, respectively. Compared with prior studies in the literature, we used a higher threshold to define an alert at greater than 80% signal attenuation in any of the electrodes—we required all 3 heads of the deltoid to meet these criteria to qualify as a positive alert—in order to decrease the amount of noise and false positives.

In our experience, when an alert occurs, there is a surgical pause, retractors are removed, and the arm is returned to normal, removing any direct and indirect causes of nerve stress that

may be occurring. As the surgeon proceeds with the case, he is aware of the decreased neurologic endurance in this specific patient and makes sure to avoid any aggressive range of motion, retractor use, or dissection. In fact, this is how we advise IONM data be utilized—similar to any intraoperative measure such as pulse oximeter or blood pressure, changes will occur throughout the case, and when a low threshold is met, attention is given to search for potential issues, and interventions may follow. In addition, as mentioned previously, different combinations of arm range of motion with or without retractor use elicit stress on the brachial plexus; having IONM screening for any alerts can provide an extra layer of protection and peace of mind to the surgeon. Lastly, IONM may be even more appropriate in the revision setting where distorted anatomy makes the case technically more difficult.

MANAGEMENT

Understanding and knowing the causes can help guide treatment should a nerve injury manifest after a TSA. The precise cause of nerve injury may never be fully elucidated, but in some cases a prompt diagnosis and intervention may contribute to a better prognosis.[11,33] Management begins with a thorough examination in the postoperative period, given that many patients may be unaware of neurologic deficits secondary to pain and functional limitations from surgery or continued effects of regional anesthesia.[14] Physical examination, review of intraoperative activity, and assessment of postoperative imaging are necessary. Patients who seem to manifest a postoperative nerve injury can be evaluated with electrodiagnostic studies including EMG and nerve conduction studies. These modalities may contribute to a better understanding of the location and severity of injury, ultimately allowing for improved prognostication and planning of interventions.[44–46] Electrodiagnostic studies usually are not to be performed any earlier than 3 weeks after suspected nerve injury, as Wallerian degeneration occurs at 10 to 14 days and 3 to 6 weeks in the proximal and distal muscles, respectively.[46–48] Hence, inappropriately early testing can miss nerve lesions, while also not allowing for any reinnervation that may occur during this time period to better appreciate prognosis.[46]

Management of nerve injuries depends on cause, duration of symptomology, and risk-benefit profile of interventions. For high-grade, neurotmesis type injuries, primary end-to-end, neurorrhaphy or nerve reconstruction with a tension-free graft should be performed as soon as possible. It is often unclear if a nerve laceration has occurred during the index surgery and a difficult decision may be necessary related to early exploration or observation in the immediate postoperative period. Delaying repair or reconstruction may exacerbate end organ changes that can happen within the motor end-plates or within the muscle itself. But alternatively, an early surgical exploration for a neuropraxia or low-grade axonotmesis injury may subject the patient to a surgery for which the natural history is favorable. If a nerve transection is discovered at time of exploration, often an end-to-end, tension-free neurorrhaphy is not possible due to retraction from the zone of injury, and grafting, nerve conduits, or transfers can be considered.[28] Nerve transfers have been shown to be an effective tool to reinnervate denervated muscles especially at the shoulder and elbow and may have a role if nerve injury occurs during TSA.[28] In the setting of suprascapular nerve injury secondary to baseplate screw placement from rTSA, screw removal with neurolysis can be performed in patients with persistent pain.[49] Reconstruction of the suprascapular nerve should be performed in patients with ER deficits following aTSA.[33]

Most iatrogenic nerve injuries after TSA are generally treated with observation, as many are neuropraxias or low-grade axonotmesis-type injuries that resolve quickly or within 6 to 12 months.[6,19] Serial clinical assessments and electrodiagnostic studies can be used to look for evidence of reinnervation and return of neural function. If no such signs are present at 3 months postoperatively, surgical exploration can be contemplated at this point considering the use of autogenous interpositional nerve grafts, allografts, nerve transfers, and muscle or tendon transfers depending on intraoperative findings.[28] These early and late surgical approaches require serious scrutiny, as their success rates may be limited particularly in older populations, in addition to added morbidity from another surgical procedure including risk of infection and instability for recent TSA. Injuries that may be suspected due to lengthening in rTSA generally resolve with conservative management and do not require revision surgery.[50]

For patients who develop DPN, typically in either the ulnar and/or median (carpel tunnel) nerves, management can follow standard guidelines for these compressive neuropathies including surgical and nonsurgical care. Nerve decompression at the expected site of entrapment may be indicated but such surgery may be considered within the context of an ongoing rehabilitative course from TSA. Pharmacotherapy is also an option for neuropathic pain with agents such as gabapentin, antidepressants, and lamotrigine.[51]

SUMMARY

Neurologic injury following total shoulder arthroplasty ranges from neuropraxia to neurotmesis that can cause functional deficits and/or debilitating pain in the postoperative period. Causes of nerve injury include direct causes such as laceration and retractor use to indirect causes such as arm positioning and lengthening. Having a strong understanding of anatomy and high-risk surgical steps or landmarks, minimizing extreme arm positioning and lengthening, and use of intraoperative nerve monitoring can help to minimize or entirely avoid intraoperative neurologic injuries during TSA. Management and diagnosis of patients with neurologic symptoms should start with electrodiagnostic studies at 3 weeks. Patients with known direct injury should have nerve reconstruction as soon as possible, whereas those with unknown causes can be managed with serial examinations and/or surgical interventions such as nerve grafts, transfers, or muscle/tendon transfers.

CLINICS CARE POINTS

- Iatrogenic nerve injuries following shoulder arthroplasty are cited at 1% to 18.7% in the current literature.
- DPN occur in 1% to 12.3% of patients.
- Thorough physical examination is required in the postoperative period to screen for neurologic injuries, given that symptomology is masked by postoperative pain and functional restriction.
- Causes of nerve injury include direct and indirect causes. Direct causes include laceration and compression from retractor use, and indirect causes include arm positioning and lengthening.
- Axillary nerve can be injured in 3 high-risk areas: inferior border of subscapularis, inferior glenoid, and posterior humeral metaphysis.
- The musculocutaneous nerve can be injured during excessive retractor use on the conjoint tendon.

- The suprascapular nerve can be injured during posterior or superior glenoid screw placement.
- IR places stress on the posterior cord, whereas ER places stress on the medial and lateral cords.
- Arm positions to be avoided include excessive shoulder extension and combination of shoulder abduction greater than 70°, ER greater than 60°, and extension of greater than 50°. The elbow should be supported in order to decrease lengthening injury.
- In reverse shoulder arthroplasty, emphasis should be placed on lateralization over lengthening to minimize traction on the plexus.
- Intraoperative nerve monitoring is an effective preventative measure that can give real-time feedback to the surgeon of impending injury in order to allow for intraoperative interventions that minimize or avoid lasting neurologic injury.
- Patients, particularly those with preoperative distal nerve symptoms, can develop distal peripheral neuropathies following shoulder arthroplasty. Upper extremity swelling and prolonged immobilization should be avoided.
- Neurologic deficits should be worked-up with electrodiagnostic studies no earlier than 3 weeks following surgery.
- For high-grade, neurotmesis type injuries, primary end-to-end, neurorrhaphy or nerve reconstruction with a tension-free graft should be performed as soon as possible.
- Most iatrogenic nerve injuries resolve in 6 to 12 months, and thus observation with serial electrodiagnostic studies and physical examination is appropriate and should show evidence of reinnervation and improved clinical symptomology.
- Patients who have persistent evidence of nerve injury should be considered for exploration with treatment via neurolysis, nerve grafts, nerve transfers, or muscle/tendon transfers.
- Patients who develop DPN in the medial and/or ulnar nerve should be treated with the standard guidelines for compressive neuropathies.

CONFLICTS OF INTEREST AND SOURCE OF FUNDING

The authors and any research foundation with which they are affiliated did not receive any financial payments or other benefits from any commercial entity related to the subject of this article. There are no relevant disclosures. All authors significantly contributed to the document and have reviewed the final article.

REFERENCES

1. Wagner ER, Farley KX, Higgins I, et al. The incidence of shoulder arthroplasty: rise and future projections compared with hip and knee arthroplasty. J Shoulder Elbow Surg 2020;29(12):2601–9.
2. Farley KX, Wilson JM, Kumar A, et al. Prevalence of shoulder arthroplasty in the United States and the increasing burden of revision shoulder arthroplasty. JB JS Open Access 2021;6(3). https://doi.org/10.2106/JBJS.OA.20.00156.
3. Somerson JS, Hsu JE, Neradilek MB, et al. Analysis of 4063 complications of shoulder arthroplasty reported to the US Food and Drug Administration from 2012 to 2016. J Shoulder Elbow Surg 2018. https://doi.org/10.1016/j.jse.2018.03.025.
4. Barco R, Savvidou OD, Sperling JW, et al. Complications in reverse shoulder arthroplasty. EFORT Open Rev 2016. https://doi.org/10.1302/2058-5241.1.160003.
5. Nagda SH, Rogers KJ, Sestokas AK, et al. Neer Award 2005: Peripheral nerve function during shoulder arthroplasty using intraoperative nerve monitoring. J Shoulder Elb Surg 2007;16(3 SUPPL):2–8.
6. Lynch NM, Cofield RH, Silbert PL, et al. Neurologic complications after total shoulder arthroplasty. J Shoulder Elbow Surg 1996;5(1):53-61.
7. Parisien RL, Yi PH, Hou L, et al. The risk of nerve injury during anatomical and reverse total shoulder arthroplasty: an intraoperative neuromonitoring study. J Shoulder Elbow Surg 2016;25(7):1122–7.
8. Walch G, Bacle G, Lädermann A, et al. Do the indications, results, and complications of reverse shoulder arthroplasty change with surgeon's experience? J Shoulder Elbow Surg 2012. https://doi.org/10.1016/j.jse.2011.11.010.
9. Boardman ND, Cofield RH. Neurologic complications of shoulder surgery. In: Clinical orthopaedics and related research. ; 1999. doi:10.1097/00003086-199911000-00007
10. Kim HJ, Kwon TY, Jeon YS, et al. Neurologic deficit after reverse total shoulder arthroplasty: correlation with distalization. J Shoulder Elb Surg 2020;29(6):1096–103.
11. Carofino BC, Brogan DM, Kircher MF, et al. Iatrogenic nerve injuries during shoulder surgery introduction: the current literature indicates that neurologic injuries during shoulder surgery occur infrequently and. J Bone Joint Surg Am 2013;1667–74.

12. Pitman MI, Nainzadeh N, Ergas E, et al. The use of somatosensory evoked potentials for detection of neuropraxia during shoulder arthroscopy. Arthroscopy 1988. https://doi.org/10.1016/S0749-8063(88)80039-2.

13. Esmail AN, Getz CL, Schwartz DM, et al. Axillary nerve monitoring during arthroscopic shoulder stabilization. Arthrosc 2005. https://doi.org/10.1016/j.arthro.2005.03.013.

14. Ball CM. Neurologic complications of shoulder joint replacement. J Shoulder Elb Surg 2017;26(12):2125–32.

15. Lowe JT, Lawler SM, Testa EJ, et al. Lateralization of the glenosphere in reverse shoulder arthroplasty decreases arm lengthening and demonstrates comparable risk of nerve injury compared with anatomic arthroplasty: a prospective cohort study. J Shoulder Elbow Surg 2018;27(10):1845–51.

16. Lädermann A, Lübbeke A, Mélis B, et al. Prevalence of neurologic lesions after total shoulder arthroplasty. J Bone Joint Surg Am 2011;93(14):1288–93.

17. Thomasson BG, Matzon JL, Pepe M, et al. Distal peripheral neuropathy after open and arthroscopic shoulder surgery: an under-recognized complication. J Shoulder Elb Surg 2015. https://doi.org/10.1016/j.jse.2014.08.007.

18. Yian EH, Dillon M, Sodl J, et al. Incidence of symptomatic compressive peripheral neuropathy after shoulder replacement. Hand (N Y) 2015;10(2):243–7.

19. Vajapey SP, Contreras ES, Cvetanovich GL, et al. Neurologic complications in primary anatomic and reverse total shoulder arthroplasty: a review. J Clin Orthop Trauma 2021;20:101475.

20. Fredrickson MJ, Kilfoyle DH. Neurological complication analysis of 1000 ultrasound guided peripheral nerve blocks for elective orthopaedic surgery: a prospective study. Anaesthesia 2009;64(8):836–44.

21. Wilson JM, Holzgrefe RE, Staley CA, et al. The effect of operative time on early postoperative complications in total shoulder arthroplasty: an analysis of the ACS-NSQIP database. Shoulder Elb 2021;13(1):79–88.

22. Choi S, Bae JH, Kwon YS, et al. Clinical outcomes and complications of cementless reverse total shoulder arthroplasty during the early learning curve period. J Orthop Surg Res 2019;14(1):1–8.

23. Liljenqvist U. [The natural history of congenital defects and deformities of the spine (I)]. Versicherungsmedizin 2004;56(4):174–7.

24. Rojas J, Familiari F, Borade AU, et al. Exposure of the brachial plexus in complex revisions to reverse total shoulder arthroplasty. Int Orthop 2019;43(12):2789–97.

25. Lenoir H, Dagneaux L, Canovas F, et al. Nerve stress during reverse total shoulder arthroplasty: a cadaveric study. J Shoulder Elb Surg 2017;26(2):323–30.

26. Kam AW, Lam PH, Haen PSWA, et al. Preventing brachial plexus injury during shoulder surgery: a real-time cadaveric study. J Shoulder Elb Surg 2018;27(5):912–22.

27. Marion B, Leclère FM, Casoli V, et al. Potential axillary nerve stretching during RSA implantation: an anatomical study. Anat Sci Int 2014;89(4):232–7.

28. Gupta R, Patel NA, Mazzocca AD, et al. Understanding and treating iatrogenic nerve injuries in shoulder surgery. J Am Acad Orthop Surg 2020;28(5):e185–92.

29. Leschinger T, Hackl M, Buess E, et al. The risk of suprascapular and axillary nerve injury in reverse total shoulder arthroplasty: An anatomic study. Injury 2017;48(10):2042–9.

30. Vance DD, O'Donnell JA, Baldwin EL, et al. Risk of suprascapular nerve injury during glenoid baseplate fixation for reverse total shoulder arthroplasty: a cadaveric study. J Shoulder Elbow Surg 2021;30(3):532–7.

31. Barco R, Savvidou OD, Sperling JW, et al. Complications of reverse shoulder arthroplasty. Semin Arthroplasty 2018;29(2):91–6.

32. Molony DC, Cassar Gheiti AJ, Kennedy J, et al. A cadaveric model for suprascapular nerve injury during glenoid component screw insertion in reverse-geometry shoulder arthroplasty. J Shoulder Elbow Surg 2011;20(8):1323–7.

33. Florczynski M, Paul R, Leroux T, et al. Prevention and Treatment of Nerve Injuries in Shoulder Arthroplasty. J Bone Joint Surg Am 2021;103(10):935–46.

34. Duparc F, Bocquet G, Simonet J, et al. Anatomical basis of the variable aspects of injuries of the axillary nerve (excluding the terminal branches in the deltoid muscle). Surg Radiol Anat 1997;19(3):127–32.

35. Loomer R, Graham B. Anatomy of the axillary nerve and its relation to inferior capsular shift. Clin Orthop Relat Res 1989;243:100–5.

36. Yoo JC, Kim JH, Ahn JH, et al. Arthroscopic perspective of the axillary nerve in relation to the glenoid and arm position: a cadaveric study. Arthroscopy 2007;23(12):1271–7.

37. Ball CM, Steger T, Galatz LM, et al. The posterior branch of the axillary nerve: an anatomic study. J Bone Joint Surg Am 2003;85(8):1497–501.

38. Simone JP, Streubel PN, Sanchez-Sotelo J, et al. Change in the distance from the axillary nerve to the glenohumeral joint with shoulder external rotation or abduction position. Hand (N Y) 2017;12(4):395–400.

39. Lädermann A, Stimec BV, Denard PJ, et al. Injury to the axillary nerve after reverse shoulder arthroplasty: an anatomical study. Orthop Traumatol Surg Res 2014;100(1):105–8.

40. Shishido H, Kikuchi S. Injury of the suprascapular nerve in shoulder surgery: an anatomic study. J Shoulder Elbow Surg 2001;10(4):372–6.

41. Clavert P, Lutz J-C, Wolfram-Gabel R, et al. Relationships of the musculocutaneous nerve and the coracobrachialis during coracoid abutment procedure (Latarjet procedure). Surg Radiol Anat 2009;31(1):49–53.

42. Patel MS, Wilent WB, Gutman MJ, et al. ScienceDirect Anatomic versus reverse shoulder arthroplasty, are nerve injury rates different. Semin Arthroplast JSES 2021;30(4):315–25.

43. Patel MS, Wilent WB, Gutman MJ, et al. Incidence of peripheral nerve injury in revision total shoulder arthroplasty : an intraoperative nerve monitoring study. J Shoulder Elbow Surg 2021;2020:1–10.

44. Bergquist ER, Hammert WC. Timing and appropriate use of electrodiagnostic studies. Hand Clin 2013;29(3):363–70.

45. Daube JR, Rubin DI. Needle electromyography. Muscle Nerve 2009;39(2):244–70.

46. Robinson LR. How electrodiagnosis predicts clinical outcome of focal peripheral nerve lesions. Muscle Nerve 2015;52(3):321–33.

47. Noland SS, Bishop AT, Spinner RJ, et al. Adult Traumatic Brachial Plexus Injuries. J Am Acad Orthop Surg 2019;27(19):705–16.

48. Visser CP, Tavy DL, Coene LN, et al. Electromyographic findings in shoulder dislocations and fractures of the proximal humerus: comparison with clinical neurological examination. Clin Neurol Neurosurg 1999;101(2):86–91.

49. Wang J, Singh A, Higgins L, et al. Suprascapular neuropathy secondary to reverse shoulder arthroplasty: a case report. J Shoulder Elbow Surg 2010; 19(3):e5–8.

50. Rahmi H, Jawa A. Management of complications after revision shoulder arthroplasty. Curr Rev Musculoskelet Med 2015;8(1):98–106.

51. Vranken JH. Mechanisms and treatment of neuropathic pain. Cent Nerv Syst Agents Med Chem 2009;9(1):71–8.

Risk Factors, Management, and Prognosis of Brachial Plexopathy Following Reverse Total Shoulder Arthroplasty

Zachary Burnett, MD[a,1], Brian C. Werner, MD[b,1,*]

KEYWORDS
• Brachial plexus • Nerve injury • Reverse total shoulder arthroplasty

KEY POINTS
• Most brachial plexopathies following RTSA are neurapraxias which can be expected to resolve with conservative management.
• Monitoring arm positioning during RTSA is critical to avoiding brachial plexopathy, especially minimizing the time spent with the arm in extension and external rotation.
• Significant nerve injury involving multiple nerves of the brachial plexus or combined loss of motor and sensory function should receive early EMG/NCS 3 to 6 weeks following the injury.

INTRODUCTION

The incidence of reverse total shoulder arthroplasty (RTSA) procedures in the United States has increased rapidly in the past decade.[1] Brachial plexopathy nerve injuries make up a small percentage of the overall complications from RTSA, but they have significant impact on patient outcomes by slowing the overall recovery and return of function. Orthopedic surgeons must be aware of the frequency, risk factors and strategies for avoidance, management and prognosis of brachial plexopathy, and nerve injuries following RTSA given its expanding use in the treatment of acute and degenerative shoulder pathology.

INCIDENCE OF BRACHIAL PLEXOPATHY

Multiple studies have investigated the incidence of brachial plexopathy following RTSA. Early studies identified a relatively low rate of nerve injuries during shoulder arthroplasty, ranging from 1% to 4.3% of cases.[2–4] However, the true incidence of neurologic injury following RTSA is likely much higher than previously reported as many of these nerve injuries are transient and likely not clinically recognized or documented before resolution.[3,5–7]

A recent study by Ball attempted to identify the true incidence of nerve injury following RTSA using comprehensive postoperative evaluation and identified 22.9% of patients who underwent RTSA had nerve complications after the procedure.[6] The most common nerve affected in this study was the median nerve, involving 56.8% of the patients with nerve complications. However, 81% of these patients with median nerve dysfunction involved only the sensory component of the nerve. A separate study by Kim and colleagues found an incidence of brachial plexopathy in 19% of patients following RTSA.[7] In this study, the axillary and radial nerves were most common, involving 41.2% and 15% of patients with nerve complications, respectively.

[a] Department of Orthopaedic Surgery, University of Virginia, 400 Ray C. Hunt Drive, Suite 330, Charlottesville, VA 22903, USA; [b] University of Virginia, 400 Ray C. Hunt Drive, Suite 330, Charlottesville, VA 22903, USA
[1] Present address: 2280 Ivy Road, Suite 2059, Charlottesville, VA 22903.
* Corresponding author.
E-mail address: bcw4x@virginia.edu

Orthop Clin N Am 53 (2022) 215–221
https://doi.org/10.1016/j.ocl.2021.11.007
0030-5898/22/© 2021 Elsevier Inc. All rights reserved.

More recent studies have been able to use intraoperative nerve monitoring to identify nerve stress and peripheral nerve injury during shoulder arthroplasty.[3,8] These studies have demonstrated a high incidence of nerve stress or injury intraoperatively, ranging between 24% and 56% of cases.[3,8] However, most of these signals returned to normal with neutral positioning of the arm and many of these patients did not have postoperative brachial plexopathy or peripheral nerve injury.[8] While many of the nerve injuries identified in these studies are transient and resolve quickly, they demonstrate the close proximity of the brachial plexus during RTSA and the potential for more severe or permanent nerve injury.

ETIOLOGY, RISK FACTORS, AND PREVENTION OF BRACHIAL PLEXOPATHY

Multiple studies have reported a higher risk of brachial plexopathy in patients undergoing RTSA than anatomic TSA or hemiarthroplasty.[5,6,9] A study by Parisien and colleagues used intraoperative nerve monitoring to evaluate for potential nerve injury. They found incidence of nerve alerts intraoperatively during RTSA was five times greater than during an anatomic TSA.[9] A retrospective review recently found nerve injury in 22.9% of patients with RTSA, compared with 20% of anatomic TSA patients and 9.1% of shoulder hemiarthroplasty patients.[6] Numerous risk factors for the increased risk of brachial plexopathy after RTSA have been proposed, including traction injury related to arm positioning and exposure during the procedure, traction injury from arm lengthening, direct nerve injury during surgical dissection, compression injury from retractor placement, and use of interscalene nerve blocks.[3,6,10,11]

Arm Position

One of the more common causes of brachial plexopathy during RTSA is thought to be secondary to a traction injury on the brachial plexus due to extreme arm positioning and shoulder manipulation used for the procedure.[3,8,12,13] Cadaveric studies have demonstrated the anatomy of the brachial plexus as it relates to the glenoid and humerus explains the changes in tension seen with positioning of the arm during RTSA.[12–14] With neutral positioning of the shoulder and humerus, the brachial plexus travels near the inferior aspect of the glenohumeral joint. Therefore, with increasing shoulder abduction the plexus is stretched due to the humeral head acting as a fulcrum on the nerves of the brachial plexus.[12] However, with external

rotation of the shoulder, the nerves of the brachial plexus rotate from inferior to more anterior in relation to the glenohumeral joint. While the arm remains externally rotated, this fulcrum of the brachial plexus over the humeral head is now created with shoulder extension and tension on the nerves increases with greater degrees of shoulder extension like those typically used in RTSA.[12,15]

In these cadaveric studies, shoulder extension alone increased stress on all nerves in the brachial plexus from baseline and external rotation alone increased stress on the musculocutaneous, median, and ulnar nerves.[13] However, shoulder extension alone and external rotation alone did not increase tension on the nerves of the brachial plexus above the strain threshold which leads to nerve injury.[12]

The combination of external rotation along with extension of the shoulder has a compounding effect and increases tension on the brachial plexus greater than either plane of motion alone.[12,13] Specifically, a cadaveric study demonstrated that when the arm is placed in 60° or greater of external rotation, injury threshold to the nerves was surpassed when shoulder extension exceeded 50°.[12] Therefore, the steps at highest risk for nerve injury during RTSA include glenoid preparation and humeral preparation, both positions when the arm is typically significantly extended and externally rotated.[12,13] A study using intraoperative nerve monitoring showed similar findings as 50% of nerve alerts during shoulder arthroplasty occurred during glenoid preparation and 33% during humeral preparation.[3] Surgeons should attempt to avoid both shoulder abduction greater than 70° and the combination of shoulder external rotation greater than 60° with extension greater than 50° during all steps of the procedure to minimize risk for brachial plexopathy, or at a minimum limit the amount of time the arm spends in these extreme positions.[12]

Positioning of the patient during RTSA can greatly influence the risk of nerve injury. One method to limit shoulder extension and protect the brachial plexus during the procedure is to position the patient more upright in a beach chair position. Most surgeons prefer to have the humerus presented vertically during reaming and insertion of humeral components, but as the patient is positioned more supine, increasing shoulder extension is required to achieve this vertical position of the humerus (**Fig. 1**).[13] This places increased stress on the brachial plexus, especially when combined with external rotation.

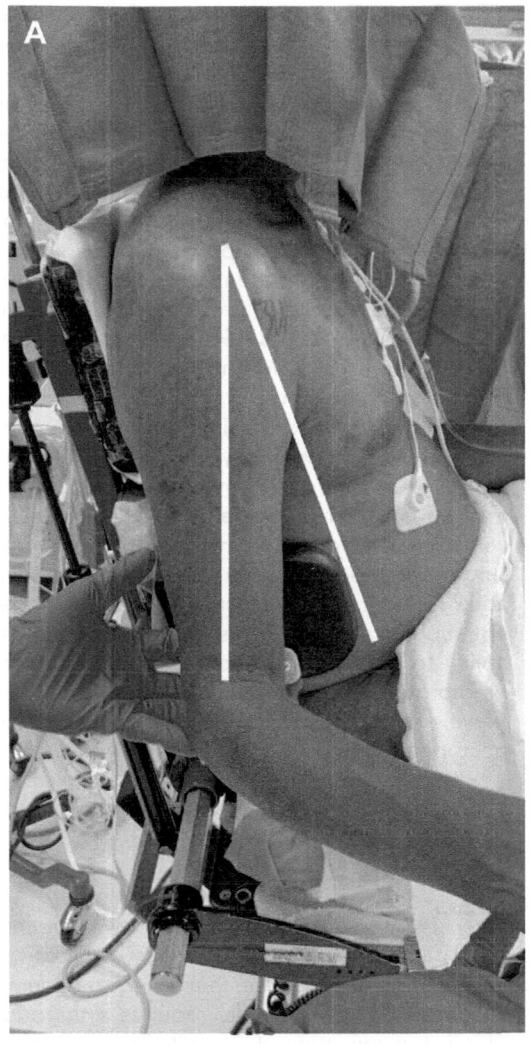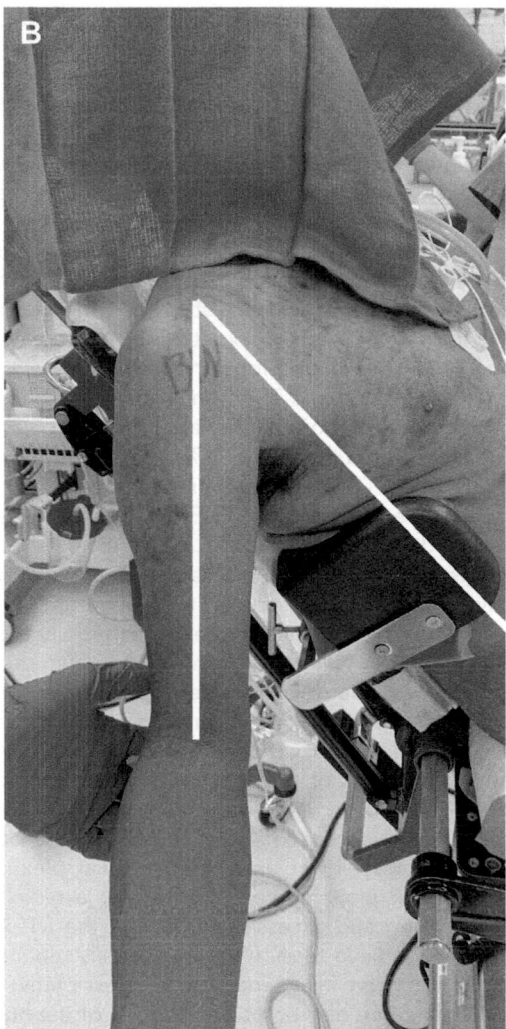

Fig. 1. Patient positioning demonstrating shoulder extension required during reverse total shoulder arthroplasty in full beach chair position (*A*) and increasing shoulder extension required with more supine positioning (*B*).

As discussed previously, the glenohumeral joint acts as a fulcrum for the brachial plexus. Retractor placement, especially around the anterior glenoid, can increase the tension on the brachial plexus even further, and subsequent movement of the arm after retractor placement may exacerbate this tension on the nerves.[12] Therefore, retractors should be removed before adjusting the position of the arm, especially if increasing external rotation or extension of the arm.[8,12,16]

Traction Injury and Arm Lengthening

Another risk factor for brachial plexopathy after RTSA is thought to be due to traction injury on the nerves and lengthening of the arm.[7,9,14,17] The nonanatomic design of RTSA implants leads to lengthening of the arm through the distalization of the center of rotation.[5,7,17] This implant design is necessary to provide a medialized center of rotation and adequate deltoid tension for proper function, but the lengthening of the arm also causes increased tension on the brachial plexus.[7,17]

A recent study by Kim and colleagues demonstrated the effect of arm lengthening on risk for nerve injury by comparing the radiographs of shoulders after RTSA in patients who presented with and without postoperative neurologic deficits.[7] They measured the acromiohumeral distance of the humerus following RTSA to evaluate the degree of arm lengthening. Overall, most patients exceeded 2 cm of arm lengthening after RTSA, but patients with acute nerve injury postoperatively averaged 4–5 mm greater arm lengthening and acromiohumeral distance compared with patients without postoperative nerve injury.[7,17]

Further evidence of the effect of RTSA implants on the brachial plexus can be seen using advanced imaging. CT scans before and after RTSA have shown an increase in strain across nerves of the brachial plexus, specifically the median nerve, as a result of distalization of the humerus after insertion of RTSA implants.[18] EMG findings have also correlated with increased risk of nerve injury with arm lengthening in RTSA. A study by Ladermann and colleagues used preoperative and postoperative EMG to evaluate for nerve injury following RTSA and anatomic TSA. An EMG between 3 and 4 weeks postoperatively after RTSA showed subclinical EMG changes in 47% of shoulders.[5] Patients with RTSA were 10.9 times more likely to have nerve injury based on EMG than patients who underwent anatomic TSA.[5]

Distalization of the humerus has been found to have macroscopic effects on the appearance of the nerves of the brachial plexus, especially the axillary nerve.[14] Distalization of the humerus below the equator of the glenoid changes the course of the axillary nerve, causing it to become straighter and more vertical which can lead to flattening and loss of the tubular structure of the nerve over time.[14] Finally, increasing polyethylene cup thickness has been shown to increase stress across all nerves of the brachial plexus except the ulnar nerve.[13] Therefore, avoiding overstuffing and excessive tension of the RTSA can likely relieve tension and potentially reduce the risk of nerve injury and brachial plexopathy.

While some degree of distalization of the humerus related to the nonanatomic design of RTSA cannot be completely avoided during the procedure, the transient lengthening of the humerus throughout the procedure can be prevented by providing support underneath the elbow in the operating room.[12] Many devices are available to support the arm during shoulder surgery and help provide easy manipulation of the arm for the surgeon. However, most of these devices provide rigid support to the hand and forearm without support extending underneath the elbow.[12] Using a device with support under the elbow or modifying existing devices would help to relieve tension on the brachial plexus by preventing distalization of the humerus during certain surgical steps, such as humeral preparation with reamers and broaches and also during implant insertion.[12]

Prior Surgery

Prior surgery to the ipsilateral shoulder also increases the risk of intraoperative nerve injury and brachial plexopathy. Prior surgery may cause scar tissue formation in the shoulder which makes surgical dissection more difficult which may place nerves at risk for injury. This becomes especially important in patients undergoing RTSA whereby more aggressive inferior capsular release is needed to aid in inferior glenoid exposure for baseplate placement. The highest risk patient for brachial plexopathy in a recent study was found to be a patient undergoing primary RTSA with a history of previous surgery to the ipsilateral shoulder as 29% of these patients had a nerve injury following their procedure.[6]

Intraoperative nerve monitoring has shown the ability to monitor for increased nerve stress and potential nerve injury intraoperatively during RTSA.[3,8] Intraoperative nerve monitoring may be considered in specific circumstances at very high risk for nerve injury, such as revision surgery or in patients with very limited preoperative motion. However, current literature does not support routine use as it has not shown the ability to decrease intraoperative nerve injuries or improve patient outcomes, as most identified nerve events are very transient or resolve quickly postoperatively.[3,9,16]

MANAGEMENT OF BRACHIAL PLEXOPATHY AFTER REVERSE TOTAL SHOULDER ARTHROPLASTY

Early identification of postoperative brachial plexopathy is imperative to optimize outcomes and provide appropriate counseling to patients. Diagnosis of nerve injuries requires a thorough physical examination at the initial postoperative assessment. When a potential brachial plexopathy is identified, initial workup usually involves electrophysiologic testing in the form of nerve conduction studies (NCS) and electromyography (EMG).[16,19] These electrophysiologic tests are important to localize the specific site of injury and determine its severity. However, EMG and NCS testing do not identify the etiology of the nerve injury.[20]

An understanding of the type of nerve injury involved is critical to guide further management and counseling to patients. Neurapraxia is the most common and most mild form of nerve injury following RTSA. It involves a block in the conduction of nerve impulses through the effected segment of the nerve but maintains conduction in adjacent segments.[20] Axonotmesis describes an injury in which nerve axons are completely disrupted but the epineurium remains intact. Finally, neurotmesis is most severe and involves complete transection of a nerve

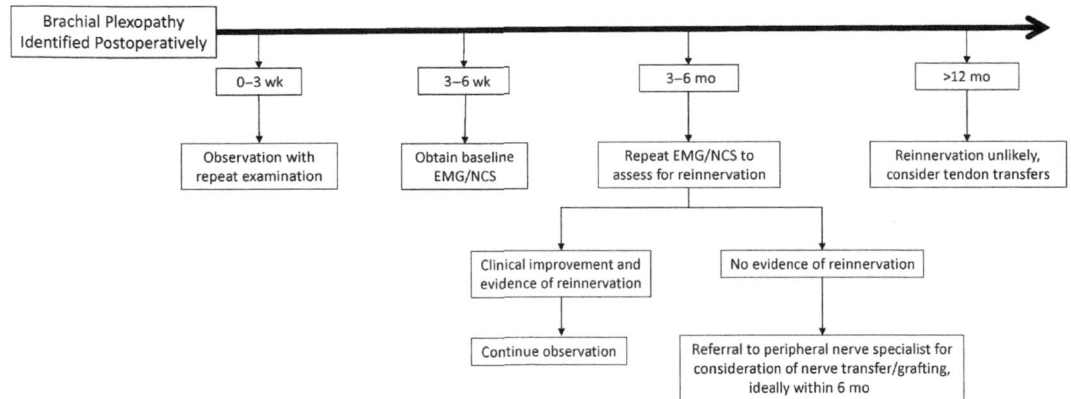

Fig. 2. Management algorithm for brachial plexopathy identified following RTSA

when both the axons and epineurium are disrupted.[16,20] Transection of a nerve acutely during surgery requires primary repair, ideally within 72 hours.[16] Nerve injuries with gaps greater than 2 cm typically are unable to undergo primary repair and require repair with nerve grafting, nerve conduit, or nerve transfer.

Given the high rate of improvement in function, initial nonoperative treatment of neurapraxia and axonotmesis type injuries has been the mainstay of treatment of brachial plexopathy following RTSA although limited studies have examined long term outcomes after these nerve injuries.[5,7] Nonoperative treatment options have included use of steroids such as prednisolone acutely along with physiotherapy with passive motion to retain motion across the shoulder and other effected joints.[7] Additionally, medical management of neuropathic pain may be used which includes the use of tricyclic antidepressants, antiepileptics, such as pregabalin or gabapentin, and serotonin-norepinephrine reuptake inhibitors, such as duloxetine.[16,21,22]

An initial EMG and NCS is typically obtained at least 3 weeks and typically closer to 6 weeks after injury as this is when changes indicating denervation are seen on an EMG.[16] If symptoms persist over time, repeat EMG and NCS at 3 months from time of injury will allow for the detection of any signs of early reinnervation. If evidence of reinnervation exists at 3 months, ongoing observation is recommended, but if there is no evidence of reinnervation on repeat EMG/NCS after 3 months, then consideration of surgical management of nerve injuries is warranted (**Fig. 2**).[16,23]

Timing of operative treatment is very important as reinnervation procedures are most successful if performed within 6 months of nerve injury and functional reinnervation is unlikely to occur after 12 months.[16,23,24] However, a prior study has shown an average of 5.4 months between the date of surgery and evaluation by a peripheral nerve surgeon.[23] Therefore, surgeons should provide prompt referrals to patients with significant nerve deficits which show no evidence of recovery to optimize outcomes and avoid delays in treatment. Surgical treatment options include autogenous nerve graft, nerve conduit allografts, nerve transfers, and tendon transfers.[16]

PROGNOSIS

The vast majority of brachial plexopathies related to RTSA are neurapraxias which can be expected to resolve over time with conservative treatment.[2,7,23] A recent study showed a 19% rate of nerve injury following RTSA, the majority of which were neurapraxias.[7] In this study, all of the patients achieved complete recovery without the need for additional surgery. The overall mean recovery period was 7.4 months from the date of surgery although patients with neurapraxia recovered much more quickly than those with axonotmesis (2.4 vs 22 months).[7] More specifically, axillary nerve injury fully recovered by 3.4 months, radial nerve recovered by 4.8 months, combined axillary and radial nerve injury recovered by 13 months, median nerve recovered by 5.3 months, and musculocutaneous recovered by 5.7 months.[7]

Another study found a rate of nerve injury in 22.9% of patients following RTSA.[6] The median nerve was most commonly injured nerve in this study, accounting for almost 57% of nerve injuries. They found patients with combined nerve injury involving more than one nerve had slower recovery which on average took greater than 12 months to resolve. 16% of patients with a median nerve injury had more severe symptoms which included motor and sensory components of the nerve. These patients had the worst outcomes, with motor function recovering in 6 to 12 months, but 3 of the 4 patients had persistent sensory abnormalities in median nerve distribution at 18 months postoperatively.[6] Overall, in the setting of axonotmesis with motor and sensory loss, recovery of motor function can be expected to occur by 6 to 12 months while sensory function can take much longer to resolve.[6,7]

Another study found postoperative EMG changes in 47% of patients after RTSA, the majority involving the axillary nerve. However, all but one of these patients had return to baseline EMG function by 6 months.[5] A study by Parisien and colleagues monitoring intraoperative nerve function found that of 17 patients with unresolved nerve alerts at the conclusion of the procedure, only 2 patients had evidence of detectable nerve injury postoperatively. These 2 nerve injuries fully resolved by 6 months postoperatively.[9] Given the rare incidence of severe nerve injuries following RTSA, most of these injuries can be expected to resolve over time. However, when more severe injuries involving multiple nerves or loss of motor and sensory function is detected, these patients require early workup with electrophysiologic studies to expedite intervention and improve outcomes.

CLINICS CARE POINTS

- Monitoring arm positioning during RTSA is critical to avoiding brachial plexopathy. Surgeons should avoid or minimize time spent with abduction greater than 70° and the combination of external rotation greater than 60° with extension greater than 50°.[12,13]

- Using an arm holding device with elbow support or modifying existing forearm-based arm holders relieves tension on the brachial plexus during RTSA, especially during humeral preparation and implantation.[3,12]

- Most brachial plexopathies following RTSA are neurapraxias which can be expected to resolve with conservative management.[2,20,23]

- More significant nerve injury involving multiple nerves of the brachial plexus or combined loss of motor and sensory function should receive early EMG/NCS 3 to 6 weeks following the injury. If symptoms persist, repeat EMG/NCV should be performed at 3 months with prompt referral to peripheral nerve surgeon if there is no evidence of reinnervation or clinical improvement.[16,19,20,23]

DISCLOSURE

Z. Burnett: this author has nothing to disclose. B.C. Werner: this author has nothing to disclose which represents a direct financial interest in the subject matter.

REFERENCES

1. Best MJ, Aziz KT, Wilckens JH, et al. Increasing incidence of primary reverse and anatomic total shoulder arthroplasty in the United States. J Shoulder Elbow Surg 2021;30(5):1159–66.

2. Lynch NM, Cofield RH, Silbert PL, et al. Neurologic complications after total shoulder arthroplasty. J Shoulder Elbow Surg 1996;5(1):53–61.

3. Nagda SH, Rogers KJ, Sestokas AK, et al. Neer Award 2005: Peripheral nerve function during shoulder arthroplasty using intraoperative nerve monitoring. J Shoulder Elbow Surg 2007;16(3 SUPPL).

4. Wall B, Nové-Josserand L, O'Connor DP, et al. Reverse total shoulder arthroplasty: A review of results according to etiology. J Bone Joint Surg Am 2007;89(7):1476–85.

5. Lädermann A, Lübbeke A, Mélis B, et al. Prevalence of neurologic lesions after total shoulder arthroplasty. J Bone Joint Surg Am 2011;93(14):1288–93.

6. Ball CM. Neurologic complications of shoulder joint replacement. J Shoulder Elbow Surg 2017; 26(12):2125–32.

7. Kim HJ, Kwon TY, Jeon YS, et al. Neurologic deficit after reverse total shoulder arthroplasty: correlation with distalization. J Shoulder Elbow Surg 2020; 29(6):1096–103.

8. Chui J, Murkin JM, Drosdowech D. A pilot study of a novel automated somatosensory evoked potential (SSEP) monitoring device for detection and prevention of intraoperative peripheral nerve injury in total shoulder arthroplasty surgery. J Neurosurg Anesthesiol 2019;31(3):291–8.

9. Parisien RL, Yi PH, Hou L, et al. The risk of nerve injury during anatomical and reverse total shoulder arthroplasty: An intraoperative neuromonitoring study. J Shoulder Elbow Surg 2016;25(7):1122–7.

10. Srikumaran U, Stein BE, Tan EW, et al. Upper-extremity peripheral nerve blocks in the perioperative pain management of orthopaedic patients :AAOS exhibit selection. J Bone Joint Surg Am 2013; 95(24). https://doi.org/10.2106/JBJS.L.01745.

11. Sherfey MC, Edwards TB. Cement extrusion causing radial nerve palsy after shoulder arthroplasty: A case report. J Shoulder Elbow Surg 2009;18(3):e21–4.

12. Kam AW, Lam PH, Haen PSWA, et al. Preventing brachial plexus injury during shoulder surgery: a real-time cadaveric study. J Shoulder Elbow Surg 2018;27(5):912–22.

13. Lenoir H, Dagneaux L, Canovas F, et al. Nerve stress during reverse total shoulder arthroplasty: a cadaveric study. J Shoulder Elbow Surg 2017; 26(2):323–30.

14. Marion B, Leclère FM, Casoli V, et al. Potential axillary nerve stretching during RSA implantation: An anatomical study. Anatomical Sci Int 2014;89(4): 232–7.

15. Coene LNJEM. Mechanisms of brachial plexus lesions. Clin Neurol Neurosurg 1993;95(SUPPL):24–9.

16. Gupta R, Patel NA, Mazzocca AD, et al. Understanding and treating iatrogenic nerve injuries in shoulder surgery. J Am Acad Orthop Surg 2020; 28(5):e185–92.

17. Lädermann A, Williams MD, Melis B, et al. Objective evaluation of lengthening in reverse shoulder arthroplasty. J Shoulder Elbow Surg 2009;18(4): 588–95.

18. Hoof T van, Gomes GT, Audenaert E, et al. 3D Computerized Model for Measuring Strain and Displacement of the Brachial Plexus Following Placement of Reverse Shoulder Prosthesis. Anatomical Rec Adv Integr Anat Evol Biol 2008; 291(9):1173–85.

19. Tiefenboeck TM, Zeilinger J, Komjati M, et al. Incidence, diagnostics and treatment algorithm of nerve lesions after traumatic shoulder dislocations: a retrospective multicenter study. Arch Orthop Trauma Surg 2020;140(9):1175–80.

20. Aminoff M. Electrophysiologic testing for the diagnosis of peripheral nerve injuries. Anesthesiology 2004;100(5):1298–303.

21. Vranken JH. Mechanisms and treatment of neuropathic pain. Cent Nerv Syst Agents Med Chem 2009;9(1):71–8.

22. Gilron I, Baron R, Jensen T. Neuropathic pain: principles of diagnosis and treatment. Mayo Clin Proc 2015;90(4):532–45.

23. Carofino BC, Brogan DM, Kircher MF, et al. Iatrogenic nerve injuries during shoulder surgery. J Bone Joint Surg Am 2013;95(18):1667–74.

24. Noland SS, Bishop AT, Spinner RJ, et al. Adult Traumatic Brachial Plexus Injuries. J Am Acad Orthop Surg 2019;27(19):705–16.

Foot and Ankle

Surgical Treatment of Foot Drop: Patient Evaluation and Peripheral Nerve Treatment Options

Nishant Dwivedi, MD[a],*, Ambika E. Paulson, MS[b,1],
Jeffrey E. Johnson, MD[a,2], Christopher J. Dy, MD, MPH[a]

KEYWORDS

- Foot drop • Peroneal nerve • Direct repair • Neurolysis • Decompression • Nerve graft
- Nerve transfer

KEY POINTS

- A detailed clinical history, physical examination, electrodiagnostic studies, and advanced imaging modalities are all helpful diagnostic tools in the evaluation of the patient presenting with foot drop.
- Acute surgical exploration and primary nerve repair is associated with the best postoperative functional outcomes, but is indicated in only select clinical scenarios such as following acute traumatic or iatrogenic injuries with a known or suspected sharp laceration to a peripheral nerve.
- In-situ neurolysis/decompression may be effective for the treatment of conducting neuromas in continuity, whereas autologous nerve grafting may be required for treatment of nonconducting neuromas or traumatic segmental neural injuries not amenable to tension-free primary repair.
- There is limited evidence supporting the use of nerve transfers for the management of foot-drop.

INTRODUCTION/BACKGROUND

Foot drop is a common clinical condition which presents with both sensory deficits and weakness or complete paralysis of ankle dorsiflexion. Patients with foot drop may also present with weakness of the lateral and/or posterior compartments of the leg depending on the location of the pathologic neural lesion. Foot drop is associated with substantial gait abnormalities and a significant increase in the risk of falls and injury.[1,2] The pathophysiology of foot drop is diverse and may be multifactorial in nature. The most common etiology of foot drop is peripheral compression of the common peroneal nerve (CPN), responsible for innervating the tibialis anterior—the primary dorsiflexor of the foot.[1,2] However, foot drop may also occur secondary to peripheral nerve lesions distal or proximal to the level of the CPN.

Effective surgical management of foot drop is highly dependent on the mechanism of initial injury, the duration of clinical symptoms, the severity of neural injury, and the capacity for spontaneous recovery. This review will provide an overview of the surgical nerve repair and reconstructive treatment options available for the management of foot drop as well as their associated clinical outcomes.

---

[a] Department of Orthopaedic Surgery, Washington University School of Medicine, Campus Box 8233, 660 South Euclid Avenue, Saint Louis, Missouri 63110, USA; [b] Georgetown University School of Medicine, Washington, DC 20007, USA

[1] Present address: 3400 S. Clark Street, Apartment 731, Arlington, VA 22202.
[2] Present address: 2207 Westerly Court, Chesterfield, MO 63017.
* Corresponding author.
E-mail address: ndwivedi@wustl.edu

Orthop Clin N Am 53 (2022) 223–234
https://doi.org/10.1016/j.ocl.2021.11.008
0030-5898/22/© 2021 Elsevier Inc. All rights reserved.

ETIOLOGIES OF FOOT DROP

Traumatic peripheral nerve injuries are common causes of foot drop. Acute neural injuries may occur secondary to blunt contusions, stretch/traction injuries, crushing injuries, and sharp lacerations due to penetrating trauma. The mechanism of injury and associated zone of neural injury have significant implications for the capacity for spontaneous improvement of neural deficits in patients with foot drop following acute trauma. Foot drop may also occur due to peripheral nerve compression at any location along the path of the sciatic and peroneal nerves. The most common etiology of foot drop is compression of the CPN at the level of the fibular neck. Peripheral nerve compression may occur secondary to soft tissue and bony masses, external compression such as due to intraoperative positioning or plaster casting, or repetitive compression from functional activities such as habitual leg crossing or squatting. Iatrogenic injury is also an important cause of foot drop, and orthopedic surgical procedures are the most common cause of iatrogenic peripheral nerve injuries requiring intervention. Nerve palsies resulting in foot drop are well-reported albeit uncommon complications following total hip and total knee arthroplasty, arthroscopic surgical procedures of the knee, and lower extremity fracture fixation. Finally, peripheral nerve lesions secondary to disc herniation or spinal stenosis, external compression, or iatrogenic injury at the level of the lumbar spine and lumbosacral plexus may also result in clinical foot drop. For a detailed description of the diverse etiologies of foot drop, the authors direct readers to the Dwivedi and colleagues' article "Surgical Treatment of Foot Drop: Pathophysiology & Tendon Transfers for Restoration of Motor Function," in this issue.

PATIENT EVALUATION OVERVIEW

Clinical History

Evaluation of the patient presenting with foot drop should begin with a detailed clinical history. It is important to determine the quality and severity of the patient's symptoms, ranging from mild sensory deficits, and motor weakness to dense numbness and flaccid paralysis, as this may influence clinical decision-making. The temporal evolution of the patient's symptoms, including acuity of onset, duration of symptoms, and change in severity over time, should be assessed. Any history of acute injury or trauma before the onset of symptoms should be elicited. Perhaps most importantly, the functional impact of the patient's symptoms on their quality of life and ability to participate in their desired activities should be assessed. The clinician should have a transparent conversation with the patient regarding their most significant functional deficits and realistic goals for recovery. Is the patient a competitive athlete striving to return to high-level sports? Or would the patient be satisfied with the ability to ambulate comfortably in the community using a walker for assistance? Establishing a mutual understanding of patient expectations is critical to creating an effective, patient-centered treatment plan.

Physical Examination

A detailed physical examination of the patient with foot drop is incredibly useful in establishing the severity of the patient's neurologic deficits and localizing the pathologic lesion. A comprehensive motor and sensory examination of the bilateral lower extremities should be performed. The lower extremity should be closely inspected for signs of muscle atrophy, Muscle strength is graded from 0 to 5 using the British Medical Research Council (MRC) scale.[3] Patients with a lesion at the level of the CPN will present with the classic clinical picture of weakness of ankle dorsiflexion, great toe and lesser toe dorsiflexion, and foot eversion with sensory deficits in both the deep and superficial peroneal nerve dermatomes. Ankle inversion strength will be preserved due to the maintenance of tibialis posterior innervation through the tibial nerve. Patients presenting with an isolated lesion of the deep peroneal nerve, although uncommon, would present with preserved foot eversion strength and normal sensation in the superficial sensory nerve distribution. Patients presenting with foot drop secondary to a complete lesion of the sciatic nerve will present with the aforementioned deficits as well as motor and sensory deficits in the tibial nerve distribution. These patients will also have weakness with ankle plantarflexion, great toe and lesser toe plantarflexion, and foot inversion as well as sensory deficits in the tibial and sural nerve dermatomes. Patients with a partial lesion of the sciatic nerve may present with incomplete motor and sensory deficits of varying severity in both the common peroneal and tibial nerve distributions, depending on the fascicular involvement of the sciatic nerve.

Focal tenderness to palpation and a Tinel's sign with radiating pain or paresthesias along the course of a peripheral nerve are useful clinical examination signs which can be used to localize a pathologic lesion. These signs should be used to examine the course of the sciatic nerve in the posterior thigh, the CPN as it winds around the fibular neck, the deep peroneal nerve along the anterolateral leg, and the superficial peroneal nerve over the lateral compartment as well as its medial and lateral branches at the level of the anterior ankle. The popliteal fossa and course of the CPN at the level of the fibular neck should also be carefully palpated to evaluate for any compressive masses. Lower extremity reflexes including patellar and Achilles reflexes should be evaluated. These reflexes will be normal in the setting of a lesion at, or distal, to the level of the CPN. Abnormally diminished patellar or Achilles reflexes are suggestive of a lower motor neuron lesion proximal to the CPN, such as at the level of the sciatic nerve or the lumbosacral plexus involving the L4 and/or S1 nerve roots. Lower extremity hyperreflexia or other long tract signs such as pathologic clonus or an abnormal Babinski should raise high suspicion for an upper motor neuron lesion affecting the central neural axis. Finally, the patient should be asked to ambulate for evaluation of gait. The ability to actively dorsiflex one's ankle to neutral is critical in achieving foot clearance during gait. Additionally, eccentric contraction of the ankle dorsiflexors following heel-strike allows for the controlled return of the forefoot to the ground during normal walking gait. Patients presenting with complete foot drop may demonstrate the characteristic slap gait during ambulation, with the forefoot uncontrollably striking the ground following heel-strike. These patients may also demonstrate a characteristic steppage gait with compensatory hyperflexion of the hip and knee to achieve foot clearance during swing-through phase of ambulation.

Patients with foot drop may pose a diagnostic challenge due to their wide spectrum of clinical presentation. Patients may present with highly variable lower extremity motor and sensory deficits dependent on both the location and severity of the pathologic lesion. All patients with foot drop should undergo a detailed clinical examination, and in the setting of uncertainty regarding the location of the lesion or disease severity, further diagnostic tests may be necessary.

Electromyography/Nerve Conduction Study

Following a detailed history and physical examination, electrodiagnostic studies by both needle electromyography (EMG) and nerve conduction study (NCS) are valuable tools that assist with localization of the neural lesion and zone of injury, evaluation of injury severity, and

monitoring for nerve recovery. EMG assesses a nerve's resting membrane potential and electrical response to a stimulus, while NCS assesses the integrity and conductive ability of a nerve. These studies are particularly helpful when evaluating potential etiologies of foot drop apart from CPN injury at the level of the fibular neck. It is important to perform EMG and NCS studies within the distributions of the CPN, L4-S2 nerve roots, lumbosacral plexus, and sciatic nerve to accurately localize the site of the injury; thus, the dorsiflexors and evertors of the foot, extensors of the toes, gastrocnemius, tibialis posterior, hamstring, short head of the biceps femoris, and gluteal muscles should be tested.[1] Electrodiagnostic studies may also be performed every 6 to 12 weeks following initial diagnosis to monitor for axonal regeneration and nerve recovery.

Baseline electrodiagnostic testing should be performed in all patients presenting with new-onset foot drop. In cases of foot drop resulting from acute traumatic injury, delayed testing should occur 4 to 6 weeks following the traumatic event. EMG/NCS testing earlier than 4 weeks following initial injury may result in false negative study results as Wallerian degeneration is not complete until approximately 3 weeks postinjury.[4,5] Repeat testing is particularly helpful in cases of axonal loss whereby electrodiagnostic studies may reveal increased nerve activity and motor unit recruitment before clinical signs of recovery are evident. In this instance, repeat testing should be performed every 6 to 12 weeks to monitor for improvement.

Latency, nerve conduction velocity (NCV), and amplitude are the 3 primary measures of nerve function assessed by NCS. Latency and NCV provide insight into the integrity of the myelin sheath surrounding the axon, while amplitude reflects the number of viable, conducting axons within the nerve. These parameters are directly influenced by the nature and severity of the neural injury. In neurapraxic injuries, NCS will reveal delayed distal latencies and NCVs with amplitude unaffected. Conversely, axonotmetic injuries will demonstrate decreased amplitudes on NCS due to axonal loss. In addition to these three parameters, analysis of the resulting sensory nerve action potentials (SNAPs) and compound motor action potentials (CMAPs) include examination of both the duration and shape of these waveforms. SNAP duration reflects synchrony of conduction through individual nerve fibers, whereas CMAP also reflects conduction through contraction of the muscle fibers.[4,5]

Assessment of EMG involves examining activity at three phases: insertional activity, resting phase, and activation phase. In the first 3 weeks following nerve injury when Wallerian degeneration is occurring, EMG will show increased insertional activity secondary to a hyperexcitable membrane. The resting phase will also demonstrate features of hypersensitivity in the form of fibrillation potentials and positive sharp wave potentials due to spontaneous depolarization. Active denervation will reveal prominent fibrillation and positive sharp wave potentials. Features of hypersensitivity in the resting phase can be observed within days following the nerve injury and can last for months thereafter. Motor unit action potentials (MUAPs) are analyzed in the activation phase and provide significant insight into both the nature and severity of the neural injury. In neurotmetic injuries, MUAPs will be completely absent whereas in axonotmetic injuries MUPAs may be absent or decreased. The amplitude and duration of the waveform also provides insight into the timing of the injury. Subacute injuries are associated with increased MUAP duration, while chronic injuries are associated with increased MUAP amplitude. During the regeneration phase, MUAP duration may vary while MUAP amplitude will be decreased.[4,5]

Dy and colleagues[4] and Lee and colleagues[5] have both described the principles of EMG/NCS interpretation and the authors direct readers to their reviews for further details on the fundamentals of these electrodiagnostic studies.

Imaging

Diagnostic imaging studies may be helpful adjuncts to a detailed history and physical examination in certain clinical scenarios. Plain radiography should be considered as part of the initial workup for patients presenting for evaluation following an acute traumatic injury, as well as for evaluation of appropriate implant positioning in the setting of postoperative nerve palsy following total hip arthroplasty, total knee arthroplasty, and high tibial osteotomy. Ultrasound and MRI may be useful diagnostic tools for the assessment of perineural scarring, focal nerve enlargement, and nerve continuity in the setting of traumatic or iatrogenic injuries. MRI may be used for assessment of multiligamentous knee injuries as well as for detailed evaluation of intraneural and extraneural compressive masses. An image-guided needle biopsy may be necessary for definitive pathologic diagnosis for masses with concerning features. Referral to an orthopedic oncologist should be considered

for these lesions. Surgical excision of an intraneural lesion should only be performed by an experienced peripheral nerve surgeon with a fundamental understanding of oncologic principles. Finally, radiographic evaluation of the lumbar spine including plain radiographs, CT, and MRI may be useful modalities for the evaluation of foot drop believed to be secondary to lumbosacral nerve root compression.

Classification of Nerve Injury

All of the clinical information gathered through a careful history, detailed physical examination, electrodiagnostic studies, and/or advanced imaging must be considered together to determine the location and severity of the neural lesion responsible for the patient's foot drop. In 1942, Seddon[6] described a classification system for the severity of peripheral nerve injuries based on the degree of structural disruption of the peripheral nerve architecture. In 1951, Sunderland[7] published a modification to this classification to better describe the severity and clinical consequences of intermediate-grade peripheral nerve injuries (Table 1). The Seddon and Sunderland classification systems provide useful frameworks through which to consider the prognosis of peripheral nerve injuries and ultimately guide management. Neurapraxic injuries, marked by a conduction block with possible segmental demyelination but without axonal loss, generally have a good prognosis with spontaneous recovery and should be managed conservatively. Neurotmetic injuries, marked by complete discontinuity of the peripheral nerve, carry no capacity for spontaneous recovery and require surgical intervention for return of motor and sensory function. Intermediate-grade axonotmetic injuries, marked by axonal loss resulting in Wallerian degeneration but without complete nerve transection, carry a more variable prognosis and should be monitored closely, with surgical intervention generally indicated in circumstances without spontaneous improvement in motor and sensory deficits.

CONSERVATIVE MANAGEMENT OPTIONS

Initial conservative management of foot drop is appropriate for most patients presenting with evidence of a neurapraxic or low-grade axonotmetic injury, as described by the Seddon and Sunderland classification systems.[6,7] Conservative management consists primarily of activity modification such as the cessation of habitual leg crossing or prolonged squatting/kneeling, provision of an ankle-foot orthosis (AFO) to

Table 1
Seddon and Sunderland classifications of peripheral nerve injuries

Seddon	Sunderland	Neural Injury	Potential for Recovery
Neurapraxia	I	Intrafasciular edema, conduction block with possible segmental demyelenation; no axonal loss	Full/excellent; 1 wk – 3 mo
Axonotmesis	II	Axonal disruption with intact endoneural tube	Full/good; 1-6 mo
Axonotmesis	III	Axonal disruption with torn endoneurium	Incomplete/fair; slow recovery, may be >12 mo
Axonotmesis	IV	Axonal disruption with torn endoneurium & perineurium; intact epineurium	Incomplete/poor; neuroma in continuity
Neurotmesis	V	Complete nerve discontinuity	No recovery without surgical intervention

Data from Seddon HJ: A classification of nerve injuries. Br Med J 1942;2(4260):237-239 and Sunderland S: A classification of peripheral nerve injuries producing loss of function. Brain 1951;74(4):491-516.

assist with ambulation, and physical therapy for the initiation of active and passive range of motion exercises to maintain full passive joint range of motion. Patients should be examined every 4 to 6 weeks for repeat assessment of motor strength and sensory deficits. A Tinel's sign that advances distally along the course of a nerve on repeat clinical assessments is a useful sign of regenerating axonal injury. A strong Tinel's sign that remains stationary is concerning for a nonregenerating injury and neuroma formation. Repeat EMG/NCS studies may be performed at 6 to 12 weeks to assess for early recovery of a neurapraxic or axonotmetic injury. Patients who fail to demonstrate significant spontaneous recovery on repeat clinical assessments and/or electrodiagnostic studies may be candidates for surgical intervention to regain sensorimotor function.[1,8–11]

SURGICAL TREATMENT OPTIONS
Acute Surgical Exploration and Primary Nerve Repair

Timing of surgical intervention for the management of foot drop is controversial and is dependent on a variety of clinical factors. Acute surgical exploration and primary nerve repair are indicated in only select clinical scenarios, as in most circumstances, time must be allowed for the zone of peripheral nerve injury to declare itself or to monitor for spontaneous recovery of nerve function. In the setting of an acute traumatic or iatrogenic injury with a known sharp laceration of the nerve, acute surgical exploration and primary nerve repair are warranted. This may occur such as during stab injuries to the extremity or intraoperative injuries during

open or arthroscopic procedures around the knee and posterior femur. Patients who are found to have a new postoperative foot drop after open reduction and internal fixation of periarticular fractures about the knee or percutaneous lower extremity procedures (ie, varicose vein procedures, less invasive stabilization system tibial plating) may also be candidates for acute intervention.[9,12,13] Patient who are found to have a discrete compressive mass causing their neurologic deficits may also benefit from early intervention for surgical excision following a thorough workup and evaluation of the mass. Finally, patients with CPN palsy following a multiligamentous knee injury or periarticular tibia fracture may benefit from a form of early intervention, although surgical timing and intra-operative management of neural injuries is controversial within this population. Communication with the surgeon performing the multiligamentous knee reconstruction or fracture fixation for these patients should begin early, before the patient's sentinel surgical procedure. In general, the authors provide technical assistance if requested for intraoperative assessment of neural injury and possible CPN decompression, but do not advocate for CPN reconstruction less than 3 weeks from injury as the zone of neural injury has yet to declare itself within this time period. Acute repair or nerve reconstruction is only performed within the first 3 weeks if the nerve is found to be in discontinuity, through either preoperative imaging or intraoperative assessment. A detailed description of the authors' approach to surgical timing within this population can be found in a recent review by Dy and colleagues.[11]

Early intervention should focus on a thorough exploration and evaluation of the peripheral nerve to identify the site of injury. In the setting of a partial or complete sharp transection of the nerve, the nerve must be sufficiently mobilized with the aim of performing a primary nerve repair with a tension-free coaptation. The nerve stumps are prepared with use of a number 15 or 11 scalpel blade against a wooden disposable tongue blade to identify the level of healthy-appearing nerve architecture with pooching individual fascicles. In the acute setting following a sharp laceration before neuroma formation has occurred, minimal nerve stump resection is typically necessary. There is no clear clinical consensus on the optimal surgical repair technique, although most peripheral nerve surgeons elect to perform an epineural repair using 8 to 0 or 9 to 0 monofilament nylon suture.[14–17] Giddins and colleagues[17] demonstrated that 8 to 0 nylon suture tended to pull out of repaired nerve endings and 10 to 0 nylon sutures typically failed under tension, whereas 9 to 0 nylon suture withstood the greatest distractive force. Prior studies have failed to demonstrate any single superior epineural or fasicular repair technique.[18] It is our preference to perform an epineural repair using several 9 to 0 monofilament nylon sutures to achieve a tension-free coaptation. If the nerve ends cannot be approximated without rupture of a 9 to 0 nylon suture or without gapping at the repair site, the nerve coaptation is under excessive tension and alternate techniques such as use of a small nerve graft must be considered. Following primary repair, in our practice the nerve coaptation site is then reinforced with fibrin glue,[19,20] although augmentation with a variety of bioabsorbable nerve wraps/conduits has also been described.[21]

Delayed Surgical Exploration and Neurolysis/Decompression

In the absence of a known sharp laceration or acute iatrogenic injury to a nerve, most patients presenting with foot drop will initially undergo a period of conservative management with serial examinations to assess for spontaneous recovery of nerve function. Delayed surgical intervention for exploration and neurolysis/decompression of the nerve may be warranted for patients who fail to show improvements in motor and sensory function within 3 to 6 months. This is most commonly required for foot drop secondary to common peroneal palsy, the most common compressive neuropathy of the lower extremity.[22,23] Delayed surgical exploration and neurolysis/decompression may also be indicated

following blunt trauma, traction injuries, and crush injuries which fail to spontaneously improve by 3 to 6 months, as well as for persistent motor and sensory deficits following total hip arthroplasty and total knee arthroplasty despite conservative management. Decompression may be necessary at the level of the CPN at the fibular neck, the deep or superficial peroneal nerves in the distal leg, or the sciatic nerve in the posterior thigh depending on the location of neural injury. Patients presenting with foot drop secondary to ballistic injuries typically have an extensive zone of neural injury and are not good candidates for decompression alone. Patients with signs of active muscle denervation such as fibrillations and positive sharp waves on their initial EMG/NCS studies may benefit from early nerve exploration and decompression. Patients with motor and/or sensory abnormalities without signs of active muscle denervation on their initial EMG/NCS undergo initial conservative management. If a repeat EMG/NCS at 3 months suggests a neurapraxic or axonometic injury without any improvement in motor or sensory signals or new signs of active muscle denervation, the authors recommend proceeding with surgical exploration and decompression at that time. There is no clear consensus regarding optimal management if the 3-month EMG/NCS demonstrates signs of nerve recovery such as increased recruitment of motor unit potentials or voluntary motor units. Some peripheral nerve surgeons would advocate for decompression of the nerve at this time, while others would continue to monitor for an additional 3 to 6 months for continued spontaneous recovery. There is also controversy surrounding timing of intervention for foot drop secondary to multiligamentous knee injuries. In this scenario, the authors generally do not advocate for early exploration and reconstruction of the nerve less than 3 weeks from injury to allow time for the zone of injury to present itself. Nerve exploration and decompression with possible nerve grafting may be considered greater than 3 weeks from injury at the time of ligament reconstruction if preoperative imaging demonstrates nerve discontinuity, or at 3 months in the setting of neurapraxic or axonotmetic injuries without significant improvement on repeat EMG/NCS studies.

Author's Preferred Technique: Common Peroneal Nerve Decompression at the Fibular Neck

The most common site of peripheral nerve entrapment or injury resulting in foot drop is at the level of the CPN at the fibular neck. Prior studies have demonstrated favorable results following surgical exploration and neurolysis of the CPN at this level with 88% of patients recovering useful function in one series.[24] Our preferred surgical technique for CPN decompression at the fibular neck is as follows:

The patient is positioned in the supine position with a bump under the ipsilateral hip and a padded foam leg ramp under the operative knee. The fibular head is palpated and marked. A 6–8 cm curvilinear incision is made 1–2 cm distal to and centered around the fibular head. The skin and subcutaneous tissue is sharply incised using a number 15 scalpel and the dissection is carried deeply to the level of the fascia overlying the lateral compartment, ensuring to raise full-thickness soft tissue flaps. Care is taken to avoid injury to the lateral sural cutaneous nerve in the proximal aspect of the incision. The CPN may be palpated along its course just distal to the fibular head in slim patients, although this may be difficult in patients with a higher body mass index. Rather, the CPN is identified just posterior to the biceps femoris tendon within the proximal portion of the surgical incision and is followed distally to the level of the fibular neck. The CPN is neurolysed carefully along its course using tenotomy scissors. The fascia overlying the lateral compartment and the lateral $1/2$ of the anterior compartment is sharply incised. The first primary site of nerve compression that is now encountered is the posterior crural intermuscular septum. Tenotomy scissors are used to carefully define the anterior and posterior surfaces of the septum and the septum is sharply divided in its entirety, ensuring to avoid injury to any small perforating vessels. A secondary site of nerve compression may be found posterior to the CPN at this level, at the leading edge of the anterior fascia overlying the soleus muscle. If this fascia is felt to be tight and a source of compression, it is carefully divided in its entirety. The CPN is then neurolysed medially until the second primary site of nerve compression is identified: the anterior crural intermuscular septum. The anterior and posterior surfaces of this septum are defined in a similar fashion using tenotomy scissors and the septum is carefully divided along its entire width. The third and final primary site of nerve compression which must be identified is the innominate septum between the extensor hallucis longus and tibialis anterior muscle bellies, and is encountered approximately 1 cm medial to the anterior intermuscular septum. The innominate septum is then carefully divided in its entirety. The CPN is then confirmed to be completely decompressed without any remaining sites of nerve compression along its entire length around the fibular neck to the tibial crest medially. The branching point of the CPN into the deep peroneal nerve, superficial peroneal nerve, and the anterior recurrent branch is visualized and confirmed to be decompressed. If there is any compression noted of the proximal superficial peroneal nerve, the lateral compartment fascia overlying the nerve is released for 1–2 cm distally along the course of the nerve. The wound is then irrigated thoroughly and a layered closure is performed using 3 to 0 Monocryl deep dermal sutures and a running 4 to 0 Monocryl subcuticular suture.

Nerve Grafting and Nerve Transfers

For patients in which a neuroma in continuity is identified during surgical exploration, the nerve should be stimulated intraoperatively with a nerve stimulator. If a nerve action potential (NAP) is unable to conduct across the neuroma, neurolysis alone will not yield satisfactory clinical recovery postoperatively and excision of the neuroma must be performed.[24–26] In this circumstance as well as in situations when there is traumatic segmental loss of the peripheral nerve or when there is a wide zone of injury (often seen following blunt, traction, and crush injuries), primary nerve repair with a tension-free coaptation may not be possible. In these patients, interposition cable nerve grafting may be performed. For reconstruction of a mixed motor and sensory peripheral nerve such as the sciatic or CPN with >1 cm gap, the authors recommend use of an autologous sural nerve graft harvested from the contralateral lower extremity. The ipsilateral sural nerve may also be used if preoperative EMG/NCS studies demonstrate a viable nerve without any evidence of injury. Autologous nerve graft provides a structurally inert and non-immunogenic scaffold for axonal regeneration as well as neurotrophic factors and viable Schwann cells which are not present in nonautologous grafting alternatives.[8,27] It is critical to place the intercalary nerve graft outside of the zone of injury to facilitate axonal regeneration and avoid neuroma formation. Serial sectioning of the nerve must be performed intraoperatively until normal fascicular architecture is noted on both ends of the nerve stumps. Similar to primary nerve repair, the graft must be fixed to the proximal and distal nerve stumps through tension-free coaptations.

Additional sources of nerve graft for peripheral nerve reconstruction in the setting of foot drop have been proposed and include nerve allograft as well as biologic and synthetic nerve conduits. Although limited series have demonstrated early favorable results with use of these alternatives in the setting of short-gap, small diameter nerve defects, the literature base supporting their use for larger diameter peripheral nerves is poor.[28,29] The authors do not recommend use of alternatives to nerve autograft for reconstruction of mixed motor and sensory peripheral nerve defects, such as in the surgical management of foot drop. It should be noted that there is no clear consensus among peripheral nerve surgeons regarding the optimal management of foot drop secondary to high-grade axonometic or neurotmetic injuries at the level of the CPN. As primary nerve repair is often impossible for these patients, some surgeons advocate for nerve grafting for shorter gaps <6 to 12 cm while others recommend early referral to a foot & ankle specialist for consideration of tendon transfers.[1,11]

Another potential treatment option for reconstruction of a peripheral nerve defect when primary repair is not possible is a nerve transfer. A nerve transfer entails the coaptation of a well-functioning and expendable whole donor nerve, or nerve fascicle, to a more important, injured recipient nerve to reinnervate the recipient nerve's downstream motor targets. A potential advantage of a nerve transfer over nerve grafting is the ability to coapt the donor nerve close to the target motor end plate, thereby decreasing the distance required for axonal regeneration and consequently the time until reinnervation.[30] A nerve transfer also requires creation of only one nerve coaptation rather than 2 required for a nerve graft (proximal and distal), thereby theoretically resulting in only one potential site of axonal loss as the nerve regenerates across the coaptation. Although a number of upper extremity nerve transfers have become well established in the management of upper extremity peripheral nerve lesions, clinical results following lower extremity nerve transfers have not been as reliable. A limited number of lower extremity nerve transfers for management of foot drop have been described, including transfer of a motor branch of the tibial nerve or soleus nerve to the deep peroneal nerve.[31–33] Although initial evaluation of these nerve transfers yielded promising clinical results,[33] further investigations have demonstrated poor reliability both between and within centers.[34,35] Another potential alternative involves performing a reverse end-to-side nerve transfer for foot drop in order to augment a regenerating peripheral nerve with additional donor axons to accelerate target muscle reinnervation.[36] Ultimately, the use of peripheral nerve transfers in the management of foot drop is controversial and is supported by a limited base of literature with mixed clinical results. The authors do not currently use nerve transfers in our practice for the management of foot drop, although this is an area of continued investigation.

Patients with refractory foot drop despite nerve reconstructive efforts may be candidates for dynamic tendon transfers to restore active ankle dorsiflexion. The authors direct readers to the associated chapter "Surgical Treatment of Foot Drop: Pathophysiology & Tendon Transfers for Restoration of Motor Function" for the authors' algorithm regarding the use of tendon transfers for the management of foot drop.

OUTCOMES

Foot drop secondary to CPN palsy following knee dislocation has been associated with poorer functional outcomes. Krych and colleagues[37] found that of 27 patients with peroneal nerve palsy who underwent multiligamentous knee reconstruction, 35% required use of an AFO at final follow-up. Only 83% of patients with a partial nerve palsy and 38% of patients with a complete nerve palsy recovered antigravity ankle dorsiflexion despite treatment, which consisted of a combination of conservative management, neurolysis, nerve transfers, and tendon transfers.[37] Further studies have demonstrated similar results, with spontaneous recovery of motor and sensory deficits following knee dislocation occurring in only 14% to 56% of patients.[38] Younger age (<30 years) has been demonstrated to be predictive of a higher likelihood of spontaneous nerve recovery following knee dislocation.[39]

Outcomes Following Nerve Neurolysis/Decompression and Nerve Grafting

When properly indicated, the use of nerve decompression/neurolysis for treatment of foot drop has been shown to have favorable outcomes. In an analysis of 318 operatively treated CPN injuries, Kim and colleagues[24] demonstrated that 88% of patients with recordable intraoperative NAPs across the zone of neural injury recovered useful function following neurolysis. Seidel and colleagues[40] demonstrated that of 22 patients with a traumatic peroneal nerve injury who had recordable intraoperative NAPs, consistent with a neuroma in continuity,

73% had a good functional outcome following neurolysis with recovery of MRC 4 or 5 strength, obviating the need for an AFO. Thoma and colleagues examined 20 patients who underwent neurolysis for CPN palsy and found that 95% experienced improvement of at least one MRC grade in motor strength postoperatively, and all 3 patients who underwent neurolysis within 4 months of injury had improvement from MRC 0 to MRC 4 or 5 following intervention. Similar favorable results have been demonstrated following neurolysis for more proximal injuries, such as lesions in continuity of the sciatic nerve. Kim and colleagues[41] examined outcomes in 353 operatively treated sciatic nerve injuries and found that between 71% and 96% of patients with recordable intraoperative NAPs recovered at least MRC grade 3 motor strength postoperatively. Murovic[42] reported good functional recovery in 78% to 95% of patients who underwent neurolysis for thigh-level sciatic nerve injuries and in 69% to 86% of patients who underwent neurolysis for buttock-level sciatic nerve injuries, with better recovery in the tibial than the CPN division.

When a tension-free coaptation is technically possible, primary nerve repair for management of foot drop secondary to traumatic or iatrogenic injuries has demonstrated favorable outcomes. Kim and colleagues[24] reported that 16 of 19 patients (84%) who underwent end-to-end suture repair following CPN injury recovered at least MRC 3 strength by 24 months and did not require use of an AFO. Gürbüz and colleagues[43] reported that 4 of 7 patients who underwent end-to-end suture repair following peroneal nerve injury had recovered M4 or M5 function at a mean follow-up of 30 months. Similar outcomes have been reported following primary suture repair of sciatic nerve injuries resulting in foot drop, although clinical recovery seems more limited following injury to the peroneal division of the sciatic nerve. In the largest series to date, Kim and colleagues[41] and a subsequent review by Murovic[42] reported that following primary suture repair, 73% of buttock-level and 93% of thigh-level tibial division injuries recovered at least MRC 3 motor strength, compared with 30% of buttock-level and 69% of thigh-level peroneal division injuries.

If a tension-free nerve repair is not feasible or has previously failed, intercalary autologous nerve grafting may be performed to facilitate axonal regeneration. Several large series have demonstrated that outcomes following autologous nerve grafting for management of foot drop are most dependent on the length of the zone of neural injury and thus the graft length necessary for reconstruction. In the largest study to date, Kim and colleagues[24] reported outcomes of 138 patients who underwent graft reconstruction for management of CPN injury. Of 36 patients who required a graft <6 cm in length, 27 (75%) had a good functional outcome with recovery of at least MRC 3 strength postoperatively. When a longer graft length of between 6 and 12 cm was required, only 24 of 64 patients (38%) recovered at least MRC 3 strength postoperatively. In patients requiring a graft length of 13 to 24 cm, only 6 of 38 (16%) had a good outcome. Seidel and colleagues[40] reported that 4 of 9 patients (44%) who underwent autologous sural nerve grafting for traumatic peroneal nerve injuries with a graft length <6 cm recovered MRC 4 or 5 motor strength, compared with only 1 of 9 patients (11%) in which a graft length 6 cm was required. Cho and colleagues[44] recently reported outcomes following surgical management of 84 sports-related CPN injuries. In their series, 70% of patients who required an autologous nerve graft <6 cm in length had a good outcome with recovery of at least MRC 3 strength postoperatively, compared with 43% of patients who required a graft length between 6 and 12 cm and only 25% of patients who required a graft length between 13 and 24 cm. In the largest study of its kind to date, Kim and colleagues[41] reported outcomes following graft repair for proximal sciatic nerve injuries and demonstrated that functional recovery is particularly limited following peroneal division injury. In their series, a good functional outcome (recovery of MRC grade 3 strength) was achieved in 21 of 34 (62%) patients with buttock-level and 43 of 54 (80%) of patients with thigh-level tibial division injuries, compared with only 9 of 37 (24%) of patients with buttock-level and 22 of 49 (45%) of patients with thigh-level peroneal division injuries.

In a recent review of 28 studies evaluating outcomes following the surgical management of CPN injuries, George and Boyce[45] reported good functional recovery of MRC grade 4 or 5 motor strength in 80% of patients following neurolysis, 37% of patients following direct suture repair, and 36% of patients following nerve grafting. Good functional outcomes were achieved in 44% of patients who underwent nerve grafting within 6 months and 64% of patients requiring a graft length <6 cm, compared with only 12% of patients who underwent nerve grafting after 12 months and 11% of patients who required a graft length greater than

12 cm. In general, the authors agree with most peripheral nerve surgeons that autologous nerve grafting is a valuable reconstructive option for the management of foot drop in the setting of neural injuries with a gap <6 cm in length. A detailed, informed discussion regarding the prognosis and timeline of recovery following nerve grafting versus dynamic tendon transfers must be had with the patient preoperatively in the setting of anticipated nerve gaps of 6 to 12 cm. The authors currently do not perform nerve grafting for the management of foot drop in the setting of nerve gaps greater than 12 cm, and these patients are referred to a foot and ankle specialist for consideration of dynamic tendon transfers.

Outcomes Following Nerve Transfer

Multiple lower extremity nerve transfers for the management of foot drop have been described, although with mixed reported outcomes in the literature. An early series by Nath and colleagues[33] in 2008 reported favorable outcomes of 14 patients who underwent nerve transfer of either a motor fascicle of either the superficial peroneal or the tibial nerve to the deep peroneal nerve. In this series, 11 of 14 (79%) of patients recovered MRC grade 3+ to 4+/5 ankle dorsiflexion strength, 1 patient recovered MRC grade 3 strength, and 2 patients had no motor recovery postoperatively. However, later studies evaluating outcomes following nerve transfer for foot drop have demonstrated mixed results both within and between institutions. Flores and colleagues[31] reported that only 2 of 10 (20%) patients with follow-up who underwent a transfer of the soleus branch of the tibial nerve to the deep peroneal nerve achieved a good functional outcome of MRC 3 or 4 ankle dorsiflexion strength. Giuffre and colleagues[35] reported that only 4 of 11 (36%) of patients who underwent transfer of a fascicle of the tibial nerve to the motor branch of the tibialis anterior recovered MRC grade 3 or 4 ankle dorsiflexion strength postoperatively, and 4 of 11 (36%) of patients did not achieve any motor recovery. In a series of 6 patients who underwent transfer of the soleus branch of the tibial nerve to the deep peroneal nerve, Emamhadi and colleagues[32] reported that only 2 patients (33%) achieved recovery of at least MRC grade 3 ankle dorsiflexion strength postoperatively. In a recent meta-analysis of 14 studies with a total of 41 patients who underwent nerve transfer of tibial nerve (n = 36) or superficial peroneal nerve (n = 5) fascicles to the deep peroneal nerve (n = 24) or tibialis anterior branch (n = 17),

Head and colleagues[34] demonstrated a bimodal distribution of motor recovery postoperatively with a mean MRC grade of only 2.1 for ankle dorsiflexion strength at final follow-up. Given the limited evidence of their efficacy in the literature, the authors do not currently use nerve transfers in our practice for the surgical management of foot drop.

SUMMARY

Foot drop, marked by partial or complete lower extremity sensorimotor palsy resulting in weakness with ankle dorsiflexion, is a common condition with a wide spectrum of clinical presentation. Underlying etiologies of foot drop are diverse in nature and a detailed clinical history and physical examination are critical in understanding the pathophysiology of foot drop and the capacity for spontaneous neural recovery. Electrodiagnostic studies are useful tools in determining injury severity, evaluating for signs of active muscle denervation, and actively monitoring for signs of spontaneous neural recovery. Initial treatment options for most cases of foot drop entail conservative measures including activity modification, functional bracing, and physical therapy to maintain passive joint range of motion. Surgical nerve repair and reconstructive options for foot drop are diverse and depend largely on the mechanism and zone of neural injury, the time elapsed since onset of symptoms, and the degree of spontaneous recovery of motor, and sensory deficits. Acute surgical exploration and primary nerve repair are indicated in the setting of acute penetrating trauma and sharp lacerations of a peripheral nerve. Functional outcomes are favorable following neurolysis alone or nerve reconstruction with an autologous nerve graft <6 to 12 cm in length, while outcomes following reconstruction with an autologous graft greater than 12 cm in length are comparatively poor. Although allogeneic, bioartificial, and synthetic nerve graft alternatives are available commercially, the authors do not recommend their use for the treatment of mixed sensorimotor peripheral nerve lesions resulting in foot drop. Nerve transfers are effective reconstructive options for upper extremity peripheral nerve lesions, but the evidence supporting their use in the lower extremity is limited, and the authors do not currently use nerve transfers for the management of foot drop. Dynamic tendon transfers are indicated for patients with refractory, severe foot drop with adequate tibial nerve motor function.

CLINICS CARE POINTS

- A detailed clinical history in patients presenting with foot drop is essential and should elicit the mechanism of injury, the severity of sensorimotor deficits, the duration of symptoms, and the degree of spontaneous recovery since symptom.

- A comprehensive motor and sensory physical examination is critical and special attention should be paid to muscle strength testing and detection of any tibial nerve deficits (most often indicating a level of injury proximal to the knee and potentially limiting options for dynamic tendon transfer) and an advancing Tinel's sign (suggestive of axonal regeneration).

- EMG/NCS studies are useful diagnostic tools and should be performed at least 4 to 6 weeks following an acute traumatic injury. Neurapraxic injuries demonstrate prolonged sensory/motor latencies and/or conduction velocities without decreased amplitudes, while axonotmetic and neurotmetic injuries demonstrate diminished amplitudes consistent with axonal loss. Fibrillations and positive sharp waves are indicators of active muscle denervation. Absent MUAPs are suggestive of neurotmetic or high-grade axonotmetic injuries.

- Indications for acute exploration and primary nerve repair for foot drop include known sharp peripheral nerve lacerations secondary to acute trauma or iatrogenic injury and new, severe postoperative deficits.

- Neurolysis alone is indicated for neuromas in continuity capable of conducting NAPs across the zone of injury, while autologous nerve grafting must be performed for nonconducting neuromas or segmental nerve loss.

- In the setting of CPN palsy following multiligamentous knee injury, early communication with the surgeon performing the knee reconstruction is essential. If requested, the authors provide technical assistance for intra-operative assessment of neural injury and possible CPN decompression, but do not advocate for CPN reconstruction less than 3 weeks from injury as the zone of neural injury has yet to declare itself within this time period.

- Patients with a zone of injury >6 to 12 cm or presenting greater than 12 mo from the onset of foot drop should be strongly considered for dynamic tendon transfers rather than nerve reconstruction.

DISCLOSURE

One author (J.E. Johnson) is a consultant for Arthrex and Stryker and has equity in CrossRoads Medical, but has no financial conflicts of interest with this topic. The other authors have nothing to disclose.

REFERENCES

1. Stewart JD. Foot drop: where, why and what to do? Pract Neurol 2008;8(3):158–69.
2. Poage C, Roth C, Scott B. Peroneal Nerve Palsy: Evaluation and Management. J Am Acad Orthop Surg 2016;24(1):1–10.
3. Medical Research Council; Nerve Injuries Research Committee. Aids to the investigation of the peripheral nervous system. London: His Majesty's Stationery Office; 1942.
4. Dy CJ, Colorado BS, Landau AJ, et al. Interpretation of Electrodiagnostic Studies: How to Apply It to the Practice of Orthopaedic Surgery. J Am Acad Orthop Surg 2021. https://doi.org/10.5435/JAAOS-D-20-00322.
5. Lee DH, Claussen GC, Oh S. Clinical nerve conduction and needle electromyography studies. J Am Acad Orthop Surg 2004;12(4):276–87.
6. Seddon HJ. A classification of nerve injuries. Br Med J 1942;2(4260):237–9.
7. Sunderland S. A classification of peripheral nerve injuries producing loss of function. Brain 1951;74(4):491 516.
8. Mook WR, Ligh CA, Moorman CT 3rd, et al. Nerve injury complicating multiligament knee injury: current concepts and treatment algorithm. J Am Acad Orthop Surg 2013;21(6):343–54.
9. Pulos N, Shin EH, Spinner RJ, et al. Management of iatrogenic nerve injuries. J Am Acad Orthop Surg 2019;27(18):e838–48.
10. Garg B, Poage C. Peroneal nerve palsy: evaluation and management. J Am Acad Orthop Surg 2016;24(5):e49.
11. Dy CJ, Inclan PM, Matava MJ, et al. Current concepts review: common peroneal nerve palsy after knee dislocations. Foot Ankle Int 2021;42(5):658–68.
12. Giannas J, Bayat A, Watson SJ. Common peroneal nerve injury during varicose vein operation. Eur J Vasc Endovasc Surg 2006;31:443–5.
13. Pichler W, Grechenig W, Tesch NP, et al. The risk of iatrogenic injury to the deep peroneal nerve in minimally invasive osteosynthesis of the tibia with the less invasive stabilisation system: A cadaver study. J Bone Joint Surg Br 2009;91:385–7.
14. Rowshan K, Jones NF, gupta R. Current Surgical Techniques of Peripheral Nerve Repair. Oper Tech Orthop 2004;14:163–70.
15. Dahlin LB. Techniques of peripheral nerve repair. Scand J Surg 2008;97(4):310–6.

16. Goldberg SH, Jobin CM, Hayes AG, et al. Biomechanics and histology of intact and repaired digital nerves: an in vitro study. J Hand Surg Am 2007; 32(4):474–82.

17. Giddins GE, Wade PJ, Amis AA. Primary nerve repair: Strength of repair with different gauges of nylon suture material. J Hand Surg Br 1989;14: 301–2.

18. Spinner RJ, Kline DG. Surgery for peripheral nerve and brachial plexus injuries or other nerve lesions. Muscle Nerve 2000;23(5):680–95.

19. Ornelas L, Padilla L, Di Silvio M, et al. Fibrin glue: an alternative technique for nerve coaptation—Part I. Wave amplitude, conduction velocity, and plantar-length factors. J Reconstr Microsurg 2006; 22(2):119–22.

20. Ornelas L, Padilla L, Di Silvio M, et al. Fibrin glue: an alternative technique for nerve coaptation—Part II. Nerve regeneration and histomorphometric assessment. J Reconstr Microsurg 2006;22(2):123.

21. Aberg M, Ljungberg C, Edin E, et al. Clinical evaluation of a resorbable wrap around implant as an alternative to nerve repair: A prospective, assessor-blinded, randomised clinical study of sensory, motor and functional recovery after peripheral nerve repair. J Plast Reconstr Aesthet Surg 2009;62: 1503–9.

22. Masakado Y, Kawakami M, Suzuki K, et al. Clinical neurophysiology in the diagnosis of peroneal nerve palsy. Keio J Med 2008;57(2):84–9.

23. King J. Peroneal neuropathy. In: Frontero J, Silver K, Rizzo T, editors. Essentials of physical medicine and rehabilitation. 2nd edition. Philadelphia: Saunders; 2008. p. 389–93.

24. Kim DH, Murovic JA, Tiel RL, et al. Management and outcomes in 318 operative common peroneal nerve lesions at the Louisiana State University Health Sciences Center. Neurosurgery 2004;54(6): 1421–8 [discussion: 1428–9].

25. Oberle JW, Antoniadis G, Rath SA, et al. Value of nerve action potentials in the surgical management of traumatic nerve lesions. Neurosurgery 1997; 41(6):1337–42 [discussion: 1342–4].

26. Nelson KR. Use of peripheral nerve action potentials for intraoperative monitoring. Neurol Clin 1988;6(4):917–33.

27. Ray WZ, Mackinnon SE. Nerve problems in the lower extremity. Foot Ankle Clin 2011;16(2):243–54.

28. Moore AM, Kasukurthi R, Magill CK, et al. Limitations of conduits in peripheral nerve repairs. Hand (N Y) 2009;4(2):180–6.

29. Ray WZ, Mackinnon SE. Management of nerve gaps: autografts, allografts, nerve transfers, and end-to-end neurorrhaphy. Exp Neurol 2010;223(1): 77–85.

30. Brown MC, Holland RL, Hopkins WG. Motor nerve sprouting. Annu Rev Neurosci 1981;4:17–42.

31. Flores LP, Martins RS, Siqueira MG. Clinical results of transferring a motor branch of the tibial nerve to the deep peroneal nerve for treatment of foot drop. Neurosurgery 2013;73(4):609–15 [discussion: 615–6].

32. Emamhadi M, Naseri A, Aghaei I, et al. Soleus nerve transfer to deep peroneal nerve for treatment of foot drop. J Clin Neurosci 2020;78:159–63.

33. Nath RK, Lyons AB, Paizi M. Successful management of foot drop by nerve transfers to the deep peroneal nerve. J Reconstr Microsurg 2008;24(6): 419–27.

34. Head LK, Hicks K, Wolff G, et al. Clinical outcomes of nerve transfers in peroneal nerve palsy: a systematic review and meta-analysis. J Reconstr Microsurg 2019;35(1):57–65.

35. Giuffre JL, Bishop AT, Spinner RJ, et al. Partial tibial nerve transfer to the tibialis anterior motor branch to treat peroneal nerve injury after knee trauma. Clin Orthop Relat Res 2012;470(3):779–90.

36. Kale SS, Glaus SW, Yee A, et al. Reverse end-to-side nerve transfer: from animal model to clinical use. J Hand Surg Am 2011;36(10):1631–9.e2.

37. Krych AJ, Giuseffi SA, Kuzma SA, et al. Is peroneal nerve injury associated with worse function after knee dislocation? Clin Orthop Relat Res 2014; 472(9):2630–6.

38. Plancher KD, Siliski J. Long-term functional results and complications in patients with knee dislocations. J Knee Surg 2008;21(4):261–8.

39. Peskun CJ, Chahal J, Steinfeld ZY, et al. Risk factors for peroneal nerve injury and recovery in knee dislocation. Clin Orthop Relat Res 2012;470(3): 774–8.

40. Seidel JA, Koenig R, Antoniadis G, et al. Surgical treatment of traumatic peroneal nerve lesions. Neurosurgery 2008;62(3):664–73 [discussion: 664–73].

41. Kim DH, Murovic JA, Tiel R, et al. Management and outcomes in 353 surgically treated sciatic nerve lesions. J Neurosurg 2004;101(1):8–17.

42. Murovic JA. Lower-extremity peripheral nerve injuries: a Louisiana State University Health Sciences Center literature review with comparison of the operative outcomes of 806 Louisiana State University Health Sciences Center sciatic, common peroneal, and tibial nerve lesions. Neurosurgery 2009; 65(4 Suppl):A18–23.

43. Gürbüz Y, Sügün TS, Özaksar K, et al. Peroneal nerve injury surgical treatment results. Acta Orthop Traumatol Turc 2012;46(6):438–42.

44. Cho D, Saetia K, Lee S, et al. Peroneal nerve injury associated with sports-related knee injury. Neurosurg Focus 2011;31(5):E11.

45. George SC, Boyce DE. An evidence-based structured review to assess the results of common peroneal nerve repair. Plast Reconstr Surg 2014;134(2): 302e–11e.

Surgical Treatment of Foot Drop: Pathophysiology and Tendon Transfers for Restoration of Motor Function

Nishant Dwivedi, MD[a],*, Ambika E. Paulson, MS[b,1],
Christopher J. Dy, MD, MPH[a], Jeffrey E. Johnson, MD[a,2]

KEYWORDS

- Foot drop • Peroneal nerve • Patient evaluation • Tendon transfer • Posterior tibialis
- Bridle procedure

KEY POINTS

- Patients with refractory foot drop without spontaneous recovery of motor deficits and who are not candidates for or have failed peripheral nerve reconstruction may benefit from dynamic tendon transfers to restore active ankle dorsiflexion. This includes patients with a zone of neural injury greater than 6 to 12 cm in length, and patients presenting greater than 12 months from their initial neural injury because of irreversible motor end plate degeneration.
- A detailed physical examination focusing on a thorough assessment of muscle strength of all motor groups, any clinical signs of tibial nerve deficits, passive joint range of motion, and evidence of prior vascular injury is critical when evaluating patients for potential tendon transfer.
- The modified Bridle procedure entails creation of a tritendon anastomosis via transfer of the tibialis posterior tendon anteriorly through the interosseous membrane and deep to the extensor retinaculum, with subsequent attachment to the middle cuneiform (distally) and tibialis anterior and peroneus longus tendons (proximally). The modified Bridle transfer is designed to allow for more evenly distributed active dorsiflexion force across the dorsum of the foot and enhanced coronal ankle stability, and has demonstrated excellent subjective functional outcomes in a high percentage of patients.

INTRODUCTION/BACKGROUND

Foot drop is a commonly encountered condition with a wide spectrum of clinical presentation. Patients with foot drop may present with varied sensorimotor deficits ranging from mildly diminished sensation and mild motor weakness to dense numbness and flaccid paralysis of the ankle dorsiflexors. The pathophysiology of foot drop is diverse and may occur secondary to peripheral nerve lesions anywhere along the course of the nerve roots composing the peroneal division of the sciatic nerve. In Dwivedi and colleagues' article, "Surgical Treatment of Foot Drop: Patient Evaluation & Peripheral Nerve Treatment Options," in this issue the authors discussed a detailed approach to the comprehensive evaluation of the patient presenting with foot drop and current nerve repair and reconstruction surgical techniques for

[a] Department of Orthopedic Surgery, Washington University School of Medicine, Campus Box 8233, 660 South Euclid Avenue, Saint Louis, Missouri 63110, USA; [b] Georgetown University School of Medicine, Washington, DC 20007, USA
[1] Present address: 3400 S. Clark Street, Apartment 731, Arlington, VA 22202.
[2] Present address: 2207 Westerly Court, Chesterfield, MO 63017.
* Corresponding author.
E-mail address: ndwivedi@wustl.edu

Orthop Clin N Am 53 (2022) 235–245
https://doi.org/10.1016/j.ocl.2021.11.009
0030-5898/22/© 2021 Elsevier Inc. All rights reserved.

restoration of sensorimotor deficits. This article provides an overview of the diverse etiologies of foot drop and available dynamic tendon transfers for restoration of motor function in patients with refractory foot drop who have failed or are not candidates for nerve reconstruction.

ETIOLOGIES OF FOOT DROP

Acute Trauma

Acute musculoskeletal trauma and direct isolated nerve injuries are common causes of foot drop. Acute neural trauma may occur in the form of blunt neural contusions, traction injuries, crush injuries, or sharp lacerations of a peripheral nerve. These may occur secondary to motor vehicle collisions, resulting in proximal fibular fractures, posterior acetabulum fractures, posterior femoral head dislocations, lumbar spine injuries, or iatrogenic trauma.[1] Multiligamentous knee injuries and knee dislocations are commonly seen in competitive athletes and following high-energy trauma and can result in severe common peroneal nerve (CPN) injuries with resultant foot drop.[2] In a recent review of CPN palsies following knee dislocations, Dy and colleagues[3] noted that a traction injury to the nerve can occur at the proximal CPN, where its regenerative capacity is restricted by its limited blood supply from a single branch of the popliteal artery. Although not as common as blunt trauma and traction injuries, penetrating trauma may also result in peripheral nerve injury and foot drop. Cases of acute gluteal lacerations resulting in partial sciatic nerve palsy and CPN lacerations at and below the level of the knee resulting in foot drop have been reported.[4,5] Ballistic lower extremity injuries have also been implicated as a traumatic etiology of foot drop.[5–7] Foot drop as a consequence of hip trauma typically results from injury to the lateral fibers of the sciatic nerve, which constitute the peroneal division.[1,8] Injury to a peripheral nerve at multiple locations along its course, known as double crush injuries, may also occur in complex traumas involving multiple joints.

Peripheral Nerve Compression

Peripheral nerve compression is another common etiology of foot drop. Similar to acute trauma, compressive pathology at a variety of locations along the path of the sciatic and peroneal nerves can result in foot drop. The most common location for CPN compression is at the level of the fibular neck. Nerve compression at this location can occur through a variety of mechanisms, including external compression by braces or plaster casts, sitting or sleeping in an abnormal position with direct pressure over the CPN, and intraoperative positioning in the lithotomy position.[1] Soft tissue and bony masses – including but not limited to Baker cysts, ganglion cysts, pseudoaneurysms, schwannomas, neurofibromas, and proximal fibular tumors – can cause external compression or intraneural disruption of the CPN along its course, resulting in foot drop.[1] Habitual leg crossing has also been reported in several clinical series to result in foot drop because of repetitive compression of the CPN between the fibular head and lateral femoral condyle or patella of the contralateral leg.[1,9] Strawberry picker palsy has been cited as another unique compressive etiology of foot drop in which the CPN is compressed between the biceps femoris tendon, lateral head of gastrocnemius, and the fibular head when positioned in a squatting position for an extended period of time.[10] Case reports of foot drop have also been reported following significant weight loss in what has been coined as slimmer palsy, where loss of perineural adipose tissue is believed to result in decreased protection of the peripheral nerve from external compressive forces.[1,11]

Iatrogenic Injury

Orthopedic surgery is the most common cause of iatrogenic peripheral nerve injury requiring treatment, and foot drop has been reported following multiple lower extremity surgical procedures.[12] Motor nerve palsy is an uncommon complication of total hip arthroplasty (THA), with a reported incidence of approximately 0.6% to 3.7%, with injury occurring most commonly to the peroneal division of the sciatic nerve.[13,14] In a retrospective review of over 27,000 surgical cases, Farrell and colleagues[15] reported on patient-related and surgical factors associated with an increased risk of postoperative motor nerve palsy following primary THA. In their series, an increased odds ratio for the development of a postoperative motor nerve palsy was associated with patient-related risk factors including a pre-existing diagnosis of hip dysplasia, post-traumatic arthritis, and prior hip surgery, as well as surgical factors, including use of a posterior approach, intraoperative lengthening of the extremity, and use of an uncemented femoral implant.[13,15] CPN palsy is also an uncommon complication following total knee arthroplasty (TKA) with a reported incidence of 0.4% postoperatively.[16] Numerous patient-related and surgical risk factors have been associated with CPN palsy following TKA, including the use of epidural anesthesia, preoperative valgus deformity greater than 20°, preoperative flexion contracture, history of diabetes mellitus, female gender, and intraoperative traction and compression; however, all of these factors have not been consistently supported in the literature.[16,17]

Iatrogenic injuries resulting in foot drop have also been reported following a variety of other orthopedic procedures. CPN palsy has been reported following knee arthroscopy and lateral meniscus repair, as well as open reduction and internal fixation (ORIF) of proximal tibia and tibial shaft fractures.[12] Peroneal nerve injury has been reported as a complication following proximal fibular osteotomies and improper placement of Kirschner wires during opening-wedge high tibial osteotomies.[18,19] Meyerkort and colleagues[20] reported on iatrogenic deep peroneal nerve injuries following ORIF of bony Lisfranc injuries and found an elevated risk of nerve palsy in cases requiring secondary removal of hardware.

Lumbar Spine

Finally, lumbar spine and lumbosacral plexus conditions may also result in clinical foot drop. Several different lumbar spine pathologies have been implicated in the development of foot drop, most notably lumbar disc herniation and spinal stenosis, resulting in L4-S1 nerve root compression.[21] A retrospective analysis by Liu and colleagues[22] found that L5 radiculopathy was the most common cause of foot drop secondary to degenerative joint disease. CPN palsy has also been reported because of lumbosacral plexopathy secondary to external compression from uterine enlargement in the setting of pregnancy and gynecologic neoplasms.[23–25] A recent review of 12 studies by Ghobrial and colleagues found an average reported rate of neurologic complications of 9% following lumbar spine surgery.[26] Iatrogenic nerve root injury resulting in foot drop following lumbar or sacral spine surgery may occur secondary to malpositioned grafts, pedicle screws, wires, or other implants.[26]

PATIENT EVALUATION OVERVIEW

A detailed clinical history and physical examination are critical components of the initial evaluation of any patient presenting with foot drop. Objectives of the initial evaluation include localization of the pathologic lesion, assessment of the severity of the patient's neurologic deficits, developing an understanding of the capacity for spontaneous sensorimotor improvement, and establishing realistic goals for recovery.

Imaging modalities such as plain radiographs, ultrasound, and magnetic resonance imaging (MRI) may be useful adjuncts for diagnosis and monitoring when properly indicated in patients presenting with foot drop. Electrodiagnostic studies including needle electromyography (EMG) and nerve conduction studies (NCS) are valuable tools in assessing the location and severity of neural injury and monitoring for nerve recovery. Repeat clinical examinations are essential in assessing for signs of axonal regeneration and improvement of sensorimotor deficits in patients with foot drop.

When evaluating patients for potential tendon transfer, the physical examination must begin with a careful assessment of gait, as the ability to actively dorsiflex one's ankle to neutral is necessary to achieve adequate foot clearance during ambulation. Patients with foot drop may demonstrate a characteristic slap gait or steppage gait when asked to ambulate in the examination room. The lower extremity should be closely inspected for any signs of muscle atrophy. A comprehensive and thorough assessment of muscle strength for all lower extremity muscle groups, as graded from 0 to 5 using the British Medical Research Council (MRC) scale,[27] is essential when evaluating a patient for potential tendon transfer. The authors encourage construction of an organized table, which may be used to track MRC strength in all muscle groups during sequential examinations at multiple time points. Careful attention must be paid to any signs of tibial nerve weakness on examination, which may limit options for dynamic tendon transfer. Patients with a common peroneal nerve palsy will present with weakness of ankle dorsiflexion, great toe and lesser toe dorsiflexion, and foot eversion with sensory deficits in the deep and superficial peroneal nerve dermatomes. However, ankle plantarflexion and inversion strength will be preserved. Conversely, patients with foot drop secondary to a sciatic nerve injury lesion may also present with motor and sensory deficits in the tibial nerve distribution. These patients may demonstrate weakness with ankle plantarflexion, great toe and lesser toe plantarflexion, and foot inversion, as well as sensory deficits in the tibial and sural nerve dermatomes. Failure to identify tibial nerve deficits preoperatively may significantly impact functional outcomes following dynamic tendon transfer of tibial nerve-innervated muscles such as the tibialis posterior. Finally, it is also critical to carefully assess passive joint range of motion preoperatively in order to identify any associated joint or muscle contractures. If present, these contractures must be addressed preoperatively through physical therapy or surgically through soft tissue releases and/or fractional lengthenings. If deemed necessary, contracture releases may be performed simultaneously at the time of tendon transfer and are essential to achieving a satisfactory postoperative functional outcome.

In patients with a history of prior tibial trauma such as a tibial shaft fracture, the preoperative evaluation should also include standard tibia-fibula radiographs to assess for post-traumatic ossification of the distal interosseous membrane, as this may preclude passage or limit excursion of the transferred posterior tibial tendon. In patients with a history of severe, high-energy tibial trauma, particularly in patients with a suspected prior vascular injury, a formal preoperative vascular examination should be obtained to ensure the presence of redundant arterial supply to the foot. Careful consideration should be paid in patients with only single-vessel arterial supply to the foot, as although a rare occurrence, both the anterior and posterior tibial arteries may be at risk of injury with the standard approach to the posterior tibial tendon transfer through the intraosseous membrane.

For a detailed description of the approach to clinical evaluation of the patient presenting with foot drop, the authors direct readers to the article "Surgical Treatment of Foot Drop: Patient Evaluation & Peripheral Nerve Treatment Options."

CONSERVATIVE MANAGEMENT AND NERVE REPAIR/RECONSTRUCTION

Initial conservative management of foot drop is appropriate for patients with evidence of a neurapraxic or low-grade axonotmetic injury based on injury mechanism, clinical examination, and electrodiagnostic/imaging studies. Modification of activities that may be contributing to peripheral nerve compression such as habitual leg crossing or prolonged squatting/kneeling is critical.[1–3,12,28] All patients with motor palsy resulting in foot drop should be fitted with an ankle-foot orthosis (AFO) in order to maintain the ankle in neutral dorsiflexion and assist with foot clearance during ambulation.[1–3,12,28] There are several different types of prefabricated and custom AFOs that may be used depending on the patient's comfort and severity of motor deficit.[29–33] An articulated AFO contains a plantarflexion stop with an adjustable or a dynamic dorsiflexion assist hinge at the ankle, which allows for controlled ankle range of motion and

varus and valgus stability. A posterior leaf spring AFO is a less rigid AFO that allows for passive ankle dorsiflexion and provides a small spring during forward propulsion through a flexible posterior foot plate. Custom ground reaction AFOs are typically made of carbon graphite materials and redistribute ground reaction forces closer to the knee than other AFOs, providing forward propulsion and great control with a light orthotic. Referral to an experienced orthotist is recommended for every patient presenting with foot drop for guidance in determining which AFO is most appropriate for each individual. All patients should also be referred to physical therapy for initiation of range of motion and stretching exercises to maintain supple joints and prevent ankle equinus contracture. Electrical stimulation modalities may be used at therapy to initiate muscle contractions, and progressive strengthening of ankle dorsiflexors and evertors should begin as active muscle contraction improves. Patients undergoing conservative management for foot drop should be monitored closely with repeat examinations every 4 to 6 weeks for signs of clinical improvement in sensorimotor deficits. An advancing Tinel sign distally along the course of a peripheral nerve is a reassuring sign of axonal regeneration, while a strong and stationary Tinel sign is concerning for neuroma formation. Patients who fail to demonstrate significant spontaneous recovery on repeat clinical assessments and/or electrodiagnostic studies may be candidates for surgical intervention. Timing of surgical intervention, available techniques for nerve repair and reconstruction, and associated clinical outcomes following peripheral nerve surgery are discussed in the article "Surgical Treatment of Foot Drop: Patient Evaluation & Peripheral Nerve Treatment Options."

SURGICAL TREATMENT: DYNAMIC TENDON TRANSFERS

Patients with refractory foot drop without spontaneous recovery of motor deficits or failure of attempted nerve reconstruction may be candidates for dynamic tendon transfers to restore active ankle dorsiflexion. Although an AFO brace can be effective in improving function in patients with persistent foot drop, longitudinal use of these orthoses is often poorly tolerated, particularly in young, active patients. Tendon transfers may also be considered as initial surgical treatment for foot drop in high-grade axonotmetic or neurotmetic injuries with a large zone of neural injury. In these patients, nerve grafting may not yield a satisfactory outcome because of attempted axonal regeneration across an excessively long gap (>6–12 cm). It should be noted that there is no clear consensus among peripheral nerve surgeons regarding the optimal management of these patients. As primary nerve repair is often impossible for these patients, some surgeons advocate for nerve grafting for shorter gaps (<6 to 12 cm), while others recommend early referral to a foot and ankle specialist for consideration of tendon transfers.[1,3] In the setting of irreversible CPN injuries, some authors[34–36] have also suggested a potential functional benefit to simultaneous tendon transfer with nerve repair/reconstruction compared with nerve repair/reconstruction alone. However, the surgical indications and comparative outcomes between dynamic tendon transfer alone for such a 1-stage procedure are unclear, and the authors do not employ simultaneous reconstruction in their treatment of refractory foot drop.

It is essential that a detailed preoperative physical examination be performed for all patients in consideration of undergoing a tendon transfer procedure. The donor muscle should be at least four-fifths motor strength and have adequate excursion in order to act as an effective dynamic motor transfer, because some amount of loss of motor power of the donor muscle is expected with the transfer. A detailed sensory examination is critical, and sensory deficits in the tibial nerve distribution over the plantar aspect of the foot are suggestive of tibial nerve injury, which may preclude use of the tibialis posterior as a transfer if associated with motor weakness. Dynamic tendon transfers may not be possible in the setting of an unreconstructable sciatic nerve injury associated with refractory foot drop, as these injuries are often associated with significant tibialis posterior and peroneal muscle weakness. The ankle and foot must be evaluated for any soft tissue contractures or deformity, as adequate passive ankle range of motion is necessary for a successful outcome following dynamic tendon transfer. If a gastrocnemius or gastroc-soleus contracture is present, as determined by the Silfverskiold test, it must be addressed either conservatively through physical therapy or surgically through intramuscular or Achilles tendon lengthening at the time of the tendon transfer. Tendon transfer through the interosseous membrane may also be more difficult in patients with a history of ankle trauma or synostosis from prior syndesmotic injury.

There have been numerous dynamic tendon transfers that have been described in the literature for management of foot drop. One of the earliest pioneers of lower extremity tendon transfer surgery was Alessandro Codavilla, who as the Director of the Rizzoli Institute of Logona, published numerous fundamental studies on the physiologic concepts of tendon transfers.[37] In 1914, Putti was credited to be the first to transfer the tibialis posterior anteriorly through the interosseous membrane to the dorsum of the foot in order to restore active ankle dorsiflexion.[38,39] In the intervening decades, there have been numerous modifications of Putti's original technique that have been successfully used for the treatment of foot drop. The choice of the most effective tendon transfer is unique to every individual patient and must take into consideration the patient's preoperative muscle deficits and the viable muscle donors.

In the setting of foot drop secondary to an isolated motor deficit of the tibialis anterior, with the other muscles of the anterior compartment and the lateral compartment having full strength, a transfer of only the peroneus longus may be performed. The peroneus longus is transferred through the lateral intermuscular septum into the anterior compartment, routed underneath the extensor retinaculum, and secured to the insertion of the tibialis anterior. Adequate strength of the remaining anterior compartment musculature is critical in order for this transfer to be successful, as the peroneus longus is weaker than the tibialis posterior, and the toe extensors must be able to assist with active ankle dorsiflexion.[40,41]

If there is substantial motor deficit of all of the anterior compartment musculature but the lateral compartment muscles have five-fifths strength, an isolated tibialis posterior transfer may be performed. The tibialis posterior is transferred through the interosseous membrane and secured to the second cuneiform.[42–44] The tibialis posterior provides adequate motor strength to power active ankle dorsiflexion, and the functional peroneal muscles assist with active foot eversion and confer lateral ankle stability.

In patients with foot drop secondary to substantial motor deficits of both the anterior and lateral compartment musculature, the authors prefer use of the modified Bridle procedure for dynamic tendon transfer. The original Bridle procedure has been credited to Paul Brand and D.C. Riordan for the treatment of equinus and equinovarus deformities in patients with Charcot-Marie-Tooth disease, lumbar myelodysplasia, Guillain-Barré disease, and peroneal nerve injury.[45] The Bridle procedure entails transfer of the tibialis posterior tendon anteriorly through the interosseous membrane with subsequent attachment not only to the bony midfoot but also to the tibialis anterior and peroneus longus tendons. This results in a tritendon anastomosis of the tibialis posterior tendon. Doing so allows for a more evenly distributed force across the dorsum of the foot during tibialis posterior recruitment, preventing the development of a secondary varus or valgus deformity. Furthermore, the Bridle procedure also helps to address lateral ankle instability, which is a common complaint of patients with complete anterior and lateral compartment motor deficits.[3,46] The original Bridle procedure was modified by Rodriguez in 1992 to involve insertion of the tibialis posterior tendon into the second cuneiform.[47] The most recent modification to the Bridle procedure was described by Johnson and colleagues in 2015 and entails routing all 3 tendon limbs of the tibialis posterior beneath the extensor retinaculum rather than performing a subcutaneous transfer at the level of the anterior ankle (Fig. 1).[46,48] This is believed to help prevent tethering during tendon glide. Furthermore, Johnson and colleagues described fixation of the tibialis posterior tendon into the second cuneiform with an interference screw rather than use of staples, sutures, or a transosseous loop.[49] This final modified Bridle procedure is the authors' preferred technique for dynamic tendon transfer in patients with foot drop secondary to severe motor deficits of both the anterior and lateral compartments. A video guide of the authors' preferred technique may be accessed through Learn Surgery at Washington University in St. Louis.[48,50]

Postoperative Management Following Tendon Transfer

A structured and detailed postoperative management protocol is essential to achieve a satisfactory functional outcome following dynamic tendon transfer. Immediately postoperatively, the patient is placed into a well-padded short-leg cast with the ankle held in neutral dorsiflexion. The cast is bivalved in the operating room in order to accommodate postoperative swelling. The patient is discharged home with non-weightbearing restrictions and instructions for strict elevation of the operative extremity. The first postoperative appointment is scheduled for 10 to 14 days following surgery, during which the initial cast is carefully removed while ensuring the ankle is always maintained in neutral dorsiflexion. Surgical sutures are

removed, and a new synthetic cast is applied with the ankle held in neutral. The patient is then allowed to toe-touch weight-bear on the operative extremity in the cast for the next 4 weeks. At 6 weeks postoperatively, the patient is transitioned from a cast into a removable walker boot during the daytime and is allowed to advance to full weightbearing as tolerated in the boot. The patient is provided with a 90° nighttime splint for use during sleep in order to hold the ankle in neutral dorsiflexion. This nighttime splint must be worn consistently every night until 3 months postoperatively in order to prevent premature stretching of the tendon transfer. At 6 weeks postoperatively, the patient also initiates physical therapy for re-education of the tibialis posterior tendon transfer. Physical therapy focuses on active and active-assisted ankle dorsiflexion and active plantarflexion; however, passive ankle plantarflexion is absolutely prohibited until 3 months postoperatively. Gentle active plantarflexion, as well as the effects of gravity over time, will assist with restoring plantarflexion range of motion, as an overly aggressive passive plantarflexion maneuver may risk injury to the tendon transfer until 6 weeks following surgery. As swelling and muscle strength improve, the patient is allowed to slowly transition out of the walker boot into his or her former foot-drop AFO in an athletic shoe. If postoperative rehabilitation is prolonged, it may be necessary for the patient to transition out of the walker boot into a custom-molded AFO. The prefabricated or custom AFO or walker boot is used until at least 3 months postoperatively or until adequate muscle strength allows for discontinuation of the brace.

Salvage for Global Weakness of the Lower Extremity

In patients with refractory foot drop with substantial tibial nerve motor weakness in addition to anterior and lateral compartment motor deficits, a dynamic tendon transfer is not an option because of lack of a powerful muscle donor. This may be seen in the setting of lumbar spine disorders, Guillain-Barré disease or severe sciatic nerve injuries that are unreconstructable or have failed prior attempts at nerve reconstruction. If unable to tolerate the use of an AFO, these patients may be candidates for a tenodesis procedure using the weak, but partially functional posterior tibial tendon, with the concept that the ankle will remain flexible and the tendon transfer will act as a checkrein to prevent foot drop and improve gait mechanics. The results

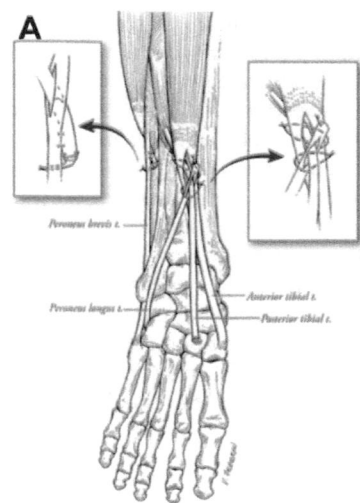

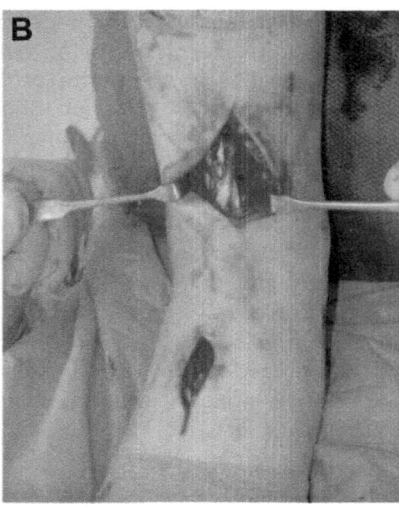

Fig. 1. The completed Bridle procedure as described by Johnson and colleagues with all redundant peroneus longus tendons removed.[46] (*A*) Following anterior passage and fixation of the posterior tibialis tendon into the middle cuneiform, the tibialis anterior and peroneus longus tendons are tensioned equally and the tritendon anastomosis is secured with sutures. (*B*) Depiction of the completed repair following removal of redundant tendons.

of tenodesis are variable and may not be durable, but do not preclude arthrodesis procedures in the future or resumption of an AFO if function deteriorates over time and is the authors preferred treatment if any function remains in the posterior tibialis, and the patient understands the limitations of the procedure.

Some authors have advocated ankle arthrodesis in order to fix the tibiotalar joint in a position of function to allow for more efficient gait.[51,52] However, without control of the subtalar joint, isolated tibiotalar arthrodesis alone may allow the remainder of the midfoot and hindfoot to continue to drift into equinus in the setting of motor weakness. Furthermore, patients with severe secondary equinus contracture and rigid or semi-rigid foot drop may be candidates for a Lambrinudi arthrodesis with or without transfer of the tibialis posterior tendon for provision of lateral ankle stability.[53,54] The Lambrinudi arthrodesis entails resection of a bony wedge from the anterior calcaneus and talus in order to dorsiflex the ankle and correct a rigid foot drop deformity.[54] The indications for ankle arthrodesis in the setting of foot drop are limited, and these techniques are not commonly performed by the authors.

CLINICAL OUTCOMES
Outcomes Following Dynamic Tendon Transfers

Although dynamic tendon transfers have been performed for management of foot drop for over 100 years, there are a limited number of series evaluating their functional outcomes

postoperatively. In one of the earliest reported series, Watkins and colleagues[38] in 1954 reported "good" or "excellent" functional outcomes in 24 of 25 (96%) patients following Putti's original tibialis posterior transfer through the interosseous membrane to the dorsum of the foot. In 1967, Carayon and colleagues[55] reported their outcomes of 31 patients who underwent dual tendon transfers with transfer of the tibialis posterior tendon to the tibialis anterior tendon and the flexor digitorum longus tendon to the extensor hallucis longus and extensor digitorum longus tendons. In their series,[55] 22 of 31 (71%) patients demonstrated "good" or "excellent" functional outcomes at final follow-up. Vigasio and colleagues[56] reported functional outcomes following a similar dual tendon transfer in 16 patients with a traumatic, complete common peroneal nerve palsy. The authors found that 13 of 16 patients (81%) were able to actively dorsiflex their ankle beyond neutral at a minimum of 2-year follow-up, and 14 of 16 patients (89%) were brace free. More recently, Yeap and colleagues[57] reported outcomes at long-term follow-up (mean 90 months) of 12 patients who underwent tibialis posterior tendon transfer for foot drop secondary to sciatic or common peroneal nerve palsy. In their series, 11 of 12 patients (92%) demonstrated MRC grade 4 or 5 ankle dorsiflexion strength at final follow-up, and 10 of 12 patients (83%) no longer required use of an AFO postoperatively. Although most patients achieved an excellent functional outcome, the torque able to be generated by the transferred tendon was only approximately 30% that of the contralateral side.[57] Rodriguez[47] and Hastings and colleagues[49] demonstrated favorable functional outcomes following the Bridle procedure for management of foot drop. Rodriguez[47] reported that all 10 patients who underwent the Bridle procedure for "paralysis of dorsiflexion" were brace free at a mean follow-up of 6.5 years. Hastings and colleagues[49] compared walking and heel rise kinetics and kinematics between 18 patients who had undergone the Bridle procedure for foot drop and 10 normal control subjects. They found that the Bridle procedure restored nearly all ankle dorsiflexion in the swing phase (6° compared with 9° in control subjects) but demonstrated slightly diminished ankle dorsiflexion during heel rise (4° compared with 8° in control subjects) and ankle power during push-off. Johnson and colleagues[46] reported outcomes of 19 patients who underwent a modified Bridle procedure for treatment of foot drop (MRC grade 0 ankle dorsiflexion strength) compared with 10 matched control subjects. There were no radiographic changes in foot alignment postoperatively at 2-year follow-up. Patients who underwent the modified Bridle procedure demonstrated decreased ankle dorsiflexion and plantarflexion strength (18 foot-pounds vs 65 foot-pounds, respectively) and reported lower Foot and Ankle Ability Measure (FAAM), American Orthopedic Foot and Ankle Score (AOFAS), and Stanmore outcome scores compared with control subjects. However, 100% of patients who underwent the Bridle procedure were brace free during everyday activities, reported their function as "nearly normal" with excellent or good subjective outcomes, and reported that they would repeat the procedure.[46] Most recently, Cho and colleagues[44] reported similar results in 17 patients who underwent tibialis posterior tendon transfer for management of foot drop compared with matched controls. The authors demonstrated substantial improvements in FAAM scores (45.7–84.4), AOFAS scores (65.1–86.2), and Foot and Ankle Outcome Score (FAOS) scores (55.6–87.8) at a minimum of 3 years following tendon transfer. Although ankle dorsiflexion, plantarflexion, inversion, and eversion strength were decreased compared with control subjects, the mean patient satisfaction score in the tendon transfer group was 94.5, and only 1 of 17 patients (6%) required an AFO for occupational activity.

Dynamic tendon transfers yield excellent subjective functional outcomes and obviate the use of an orthosis during everyday activities in a high percentage of patients. Although there are no comparative studies that clearly demonstrate superiority of 1 tendon transfer technique, the modified Bridle procedure has been shown to restore near normal ankle dorsiflexion during gait. Dynamic tendon transfers are a reliable surgical treatment option for refractory foot drop in patients with peroneal nerve injuries that have failed or are not amenable to nerve reconstructive options. Unfortunately, dynamic tendon transfer may not be possible in patients with foot drop with concomitant tibial nerve deficits, such as in the setting of sciatic nerve injury with combined tibial and peroneal division involvement.

SUMMARY

Foot drop is a common clinical condition marked by objective muscle weakness or flaccid paralysis of the ankle dorsiflexors, resulting in difficulty with ambulation secondary to poor foot clearance during gait. Patients affected by foot drop may also present with weakness of the lateral and/or posterior compartments of the leg, depending on the location and severity of their neural lesion. The pathophysiology of foot drop is diverse in nature and a detailed clinical history and physical examination are essential in understanding the underlying etiology of each patient's motor weakness, the severity of sensorimotor deficits, and capacity for spontaneous neural recovery. Imaging modalities such as ultrasound and MRI and electrodiagnostic studies may be useful tools in the initial evaluation and longitudinal monitoring of patients with foot drop. The fundamental facets of conservative management of foot drop include activity modification, functional bracing, and physical therapy to maintain passive joint range of motion. Numerous peripheral nerve repair and reconstruction techniques have previously been described for restoration of sensorimotor deficits in patients with foot drop, and are discussed in the article "Surgical Treatment of Foot Drop: Patient Evaluation & Peripheral Nerve Treatment Options." Patients with refractory foot drop despite conservative measures who have failed or are not candidates for peripheral nerve surgery may be candidates for dynamic tendon transfers for restoration of active ankle dorsiflexion. Careful evaluation of the motor strengths of all active muscles is critical for decision making about what transfer(s) to perform in a given patient. Adequate preoperative tibial nerve function and strength of the posterior compartment musculature are essential for achieving satisfactory outcomes following dynamic tendon transfers. The modified Bridle procedure is the authors' preferred technique for restoration of active ankle dorsiflexion and has been shown to result in favorable functional outcomes and postoperative independence from functional bracing. Patients with unreconstructable sciatic nerve injuries or combined peripheral nerve injuries resulting in foot drop with associated tibial nerve weakness may not be candidates for dynamic tendon transfers, and long-term AFO use or salvage tenodesis or arthrodesis may be helpful in selected patients.

CLINICS CARE POINTS

- A detailed clinical history in patients presenting with foot drop is essential and should elicit the mechanism of injury, the severity of sensorimotor deficits, the duration of symptoms, and the degree of spontaneous recovery since symptom onset.

- A comprehensive motor and sensory physical examination is critical in all patients with foot drop. Special attention should be paid to muscle strength testing, identification of soft tissue contractures, the range of motion of adjacent joints and an advancing Tinel sign (suggestive of axonal regeneration). Detection of any tibial nerve deficits, most often indicating a level of injury proximal to the knee, may potentially limit options for dynamic tendon transfer.

- Patients with refractory foot drop despite conservative measures who have failed or are not candidates for peripheral nerve surgery may be candidates for dynamic tendon transfers for restoration of active ankle dorsiflexion.

- Patients with a zone of neural injury greater than 6 to 12 cm should be strongly considered for dynamic tendon transfers rather than nerve reconstruction as their sentinel surgical procedure, as use of autologous nerve grafts greater than 6 to 12 cm in size has been shown to result in less favorable outcomes.

- Patients presenting greater than 12 months from time of neural injury should be strongly considered for dynamic tendon transfers rather than nerve reconstruction because of irreversible motor end plate degeneration following prolonged muscle denervation.

- Structured postoperative management beginning with rigid immobilization in the operating room until soft tissue healing is complete, followed by careful physical therapy concentrating on active ankle range of motion and protection from early passive ankle plantarflexion, are keys to a successful outcome following tendon transfer.

- Dynamic tendon transfers such as the modified Bridle procedure have demonstrated excellent functional outcomes and return to brace-free ambulation in a high percentage of patients.

DISCLOSURE

One author (J.E. Johnson) is a consultant for Arthrex and Stryker and has equity in CrossRoads Medical, but has no financial conflict of interest with the topic of this manuscript. The other authors have nothing to disclose.

REFERENCES

1. Stewart JD. Foot drop: where, why and what to do? Pract Neurol 2008;8(3):158–69.
2. Mook WR, Ligh CA, Moorman CT 3rd, et al. Nerve injury complicating multiligament knee injury: current concepts and treatment algorithm. J Am Acad Orthop Surg 2013;21(6):343–54.
3. Dy CJ, Inclan PM, Matava MJ, et al. Current concepts review: common peroneal nerve palsy after knee dislocations. Foot Ankle Int 2021;42(5):658–68.
4. Shevell MI, Stewart JD. Laceration of the common peroneal nerve by a skate blade. CMAJ 1988;139(4):311–2.
5. Crowe CS, Mosca VS, Osorio MB, et al. Partial tibial nerve transfer for foot drop from deep peroneal palsy: lessons from three pediatric cases. Microsurgery 2020;1–5. https://doi.org/10.1002/micr.30650.
6. Sağlam G. An unusual case of footdrop: bilateral common peroneal nerve palsy by one bullet gunshot injury. Turk J Neurol 2020;26(4):359–61.
7. Kim DH, Murovic JA, Tiel RL, et al. Management and outcomes in 318 operative common peroneal nerve lesions at the Louisiana State University Health Sciences Center. Neurosurgery 2004;54(6):1421–8 [discussion: 1428–9].
8. Issack PS, Helfet DL. Sciatic nerve injury associated with acetabular fractures. HSS J 2009;5(1):12–8.
9. Nagler SH, Rangell L. Peroneal palsy caused by crossing the legs. JAMA 1947;133(11):755–61.
10. Koller RL, Blank NK. Strawberry pickers' palsy. Arch Neurol 1980;37(5):320.
11. Cruz-Martinez A, Arpa J,, Palau F. Peroneal neuropathy after weight loss. J Peripher Nervous Syst 2000;5:101–5.

12. Pulos N, Shin EH, Spinner RJ, et al. Management of iatrogenic nerve injuries. J Am Acad Orthop Surg 2019;27(18):e838–48.

13. Hasija R, Kelly JJ, Shah NV, et al. Nerve injuries associated with total hip arthroplasty. J Clin Orthop Trauma 2018;9(1):81–6.

14. DeHart MM, Riley LH Jr. Nerve injuries in total hip arthroplasty. J Am Acad Orthop Surg 1999;7(2):101–11.

15. Farrell CM, Springer BD, Haidukewych GJ, et al. Motor nerve palsy following primary total hip arthroplasty. J Bone Joint Surg Am 2005;87(12):2619–25.

16. Carender CN, Bedard NA, An Q, et al. Common peroneal nerve injury and recovery after total knee arthroplasty: a systematic review. Arthroplast Today 2020;6(4):662–7.

17. Speelziek SJA, Staff NP, Johnson RL, et al. Clinical spectrum of neuropathy after primary total knee arthroplasty: a series of 54 cases. Muscle Nerve 2019;59(6):679–82.

18. Vaish A, Kumar Kathiriya Y, Vaishya R. A critical review of proximal fibular osteotomy for knee osteoarthritis. Arch Bone Joint Surg 2019;7(5):453–62.

19. Madry H, Goebel L, Hoffmann A, et al. Surgical anatomy of medial open-wedge high tibial osteotomy: crucial steps and pitfalls. Knee Surg Sports Traumatol Arthrosc 2017;25(12):3661–9.

20. Meyerkort DJ, Gurel R, Maor D, et al. Deep peroneal nerve injury following hardware removal for lisfranc joint injury. Foot Ankle Int 2020;41(3):320–3.

21. Macki M, Lim S, Elmenini J, et al. Clinching the cause: a review of foot drop secondary to lumbar degenerative diseases. J Neurol Sci 2018;395:126–30.

22. Liu K, Zhu W, Shi J, et al. Foot drop caused by lumbar degenerative disease: clinical features, prognostic factors of surgical outcome and clinical stage. PLoS One 2013;8(11):e80375.

23. Felice KJ, Donaldson JO. Lumbosacral plexopathy due to benign uterine leiomyoma. Neurology 1995;45(10):1943–4.

24. Dydyk AM, Hameed S. Lumbosacral Plexopathy. In: StatPearls [Internet]. Treasure Island (FL): StatPearls Publishing; 2021. p. 1–13.

25. Planner AC, Donaghy M, Moore NR. Causes of lumbosacral plexopathy. Clin Radiol 2006;61(12):987–95.

26. Ghobrial GM, Williams KA Jr, Arnold P, et al. Iatrogenic neurologic deficit after lumbar spine surgery: a review. Clin Neurol Neurosurg 2015;139:76–80.

27. Medical Research Council; Nerve Injuries Research Committee. Aids to the investigation of the peripheral nervous system. London: His Majesty's Stationery Office; 1942.

28. Garg B, Poage C. Peroneal nerve palsy: evaluation and management. J Am Acad Orthop Surg 2016;24(5):e49.

29. Eddison N, Chockalingam N. Ankle foot orthoses: standardisation of terminology. Foot (Edinb) 2021;46:101702.

30. Johnston TE, Keller S, Denzer-Weiler C, et al. A clinical practice guideline for the use of ankle-foot orthoses and functional electrical stimulation post-stroke. J Neurol Phys Ther 2021;45(2):112–96.

31. Ploeger HE, Waterval NFJ, Nollet F, et al. Stiffness modification of two ankle-foot orthosis types to optimize gait in individuals with non-spastic calf muscle weakness - a proof-of-concept study. J Foot Ankle Res 2019;12:41.

32. Karakkattil PS, Trudelle-Jackson E, Medley A, et al. Effects of two different types of ankle-foot orthoses on gait outcomes in patients with subacute stroke: a randomized crossover trial. Clin Rehabil 2020;34(8):1094–102.

33. Totah D, Menon M, Jones-Hershinow C, et al. The impact of ankle-foot orthosis stiffness on gait: A systematic literature review. Gait Posture 2019;69:101–11.

34. Garozzo D, Ferraresi S, Buffatti P. Surgical treatment of common peroneal nerve injuries: indications and results. A series of 62 cases. J Neurosurg Sci 2004;48(3):105–12 [discussion: 112].

35. Ferraresi S, Garozzo D, Buffatti P. Common peroneal nerve injuries: results with one-stage nerve repair and tendon transfer. Neurosurg Rev 2003;26(3):175–9.

36. Ho B, Khan Z, Switaj PJ, et al. Treatment of peroneal nerve injuries with simultaneous tendon transfer and nerve exploration. J Orthop Surg Res 2014;9:67.

37. Codivilla A. On tendon transfers in orthopaedic practice. Sui Trapianti Tendinei Nella Practicia Orthopaedica. Arch Orthop 1899;16:225–50.

38. Watkins MB, Jones JB, Ryder CT Jr, et al. Transplantation of the posterior tibial tendon. J Bone Joint Surg Am 1954;36(6):1181–9.

39. Mayer L. The physiological method of tendon transplantation in the treatment of paralytic dropfoot. J Bone Joint Surg 1937;19(2):389–94.

40. Cohen JC, de Freitas Cabral E. Peroneus longus transfer for drop foot in Hansen disease. Foot Ankle Clin 2012;17(3):425–36.

41. Krishnamurthy S, Ibrahim M. Tendon transfers in foot drop. Indian J Plast Surg 2019;52(1):100–8.

42. Pinzur MS, Kett N, Trilla M. Combined anteroposterior tibial tendon transfer in post-traumatic peroneal palsy. Foot Ankle 1988;8(5):271–5.

43. Hsu JD, Hoffer MM. Posterior tibial tendon transfer anteriorly through the interosseous membrane: a modification of the technique. Clin Orthop Relat Res 1978;131:202–4.

44. Cho BK, Park KJ, Choi SM, et al. Functional outcomes following anterior transfer of the tibialis posterior tendon for foot drop secondary to peroneal nerve palsy. Foot Ankle Int 2017;38(6):627–33.

45. McCall RE, Frederick HA, McCluskey GM, et al. The Bridle procedure: a new treatment for equinus and equinovarus deformities in children. J Pediatr Orthop 1991;11(1):83–9.

46. Johnson JE, Paxton ES, Lippe J, et al. Outcomes of the bridle procedure for the treatment of foot drop. Foot Ankle Int 2015;36(11):1287–96.

47. Rodriguez RP. The Bridle procedure in the treatment of paralysis of the foot. Foot Ankle 1992; 13(2):63–9.

48. Johnson JE, Yee A. Bridle procedure for the treatment of foot drop – extended (Feat. Dr. Johnson). [Video]. 2018. Available at: https://www.youtube.com/watch?v=EdG3P5Pw658. Accessed August 8, 2021.

49. Hastings MK, Sinacore DR, Woodburn J, et al. Kinetics and kinematics after the Bridle procedure for treatment of traumatic foot drop. Clin Biomech (Bristol, Avon) 2013;28(5):555–61.

50. Johnson JE, Yee A. Bridle procedure for the treatment of foot drop – standard (Feat. Dr. Johnson). [Video. 2018. Available at: https://www.youtube.com/watch?v=gulJyjo8Pf4. Accessed August 8, 2021.

51. Napiontek M, Jaszczak T. Ankle arthrodesis from lateral transfibular approach: analysis of treatment results of 23 feet treated by the modified Mann's technique. Eur J Orthop Surg Traumatol 2015; 25(7):1195–9.

52. Seidel J, Mathew B, Marks J. Bilateral ankle and subtalar joint fusion secondary to Guillain Barré-induced foot drop. J Foot Ankle Surg 2016;55(2): 260–2.

53. Elsner A, Barg A, Stufkens SA, et al. Lambrinudi arthrodesis with posterior tibialis transfer in adult drop-foot. Foot Ankle Int 2010;31(1):30–7.

54. Elsner A, Barg A, Stufkens S, et al. Modifizierte Arthrodese nach Lambrinudi mit zusätzlichem Transfer der Tibialis-posterior-Sehne zur Behandlung des adulten Fallfußes [modified Lambrinudi arthrodesis with additional posterior tibial tendon transfer in adult drop foot]. Oper Orthop Traumatol 2011;23(2):121–30.

55. Carayon A, Bourrel P, Bourges M, et al. Dual transfer of the posterior tibial and flexor digitorum longus tendons for drop foot. Report of thirty-one cases. J Bone Joint Surg Am 1967;49(1):144–8.

56. Vigasio A, Marcoccio I, Patelli A, et al. New tendon transfer for correction of drop-foot in common peroneal nerve palsy. Clin Orthop Relat Res 2008; 466(6):1454–66.

57. Yeap JS, Birch R, Singh D. Long-term results of tibialis posterior tendon transfer for drop-foot. Int Orthop 2001;25(2):114–8.

Spine Section

Cauda Equina Syndrome

Landon Bulloch, MD[a],*, Kirk Thompson, MD[b], Leo Spector, MD, MBA[c]

KEYWORDS

- Cauda equina syndrome • Urinary retention • MRI scanning • Saddle anesthesia
- Decompression • Time to surgery

KEY POINTS

- Cauda equina syndrome (CES) is a rare diagnosis caused by a compressive lesion in the lumbar spine affecting some or all of the L1-S5 peripheral nerve roots.
- CES produces a constellation of symptoms including lower extremity sensory and motor loss, bowel/bladder dysfunction, and perianal anesthesia.
- Accurate diagnosis along with appropriate timing of intervention is key for these patients in order to ensure optimal functional outcomes.

BACKGROUND

Cauda equina is the term used in reference to the collection of nerves at the terminal portion of the spinal cord and the roots of the spinal nerves beginning from the first lumbar nerve root. The French anatomist Andre du Laurens first described this structure as a tail of fibers at the end of the spinal cord. The cauda equina or the horse's tail in Latin, is the name given to describe this terminal nerve bundle that serves to supply the lower extremities, perineum, perianal region, and the bladder. In order to develop the condition termed cauda equina syndrome (CES), compression must occur between 1 or multiple of these nerve roots resulting in a constellation of symptoms. The most commonly described symptoms include bowel and bladder dysfunction, saddle anesthesia, and varying degrees of motor and sensory loss in the lower extremities. One of the challenges of diagnosing acute CES lies in the fact that the current literature lacks a formal definition or strict diagnosis criteria. The one element that physicians across the spectrum do agree on is the element of bladder dysfunction is required to make the diagnosis.[1]

INCIDENCE/PREVALENCE

CES has a relatively low incidence in the general population, with reports of approximately two cases per 100,00 patients.[2] A review by Woodside analyzed the results of 18 studies of adults with suspected CES, and found that only 19% of these patients had radiological and clinical CES.[3] These numbers overall correlate with approximately 1% to 3% of every patient who develops an acute lumbar disc herniation.[4] Acute lumbar disc herniations are the leading cause of CES, representing approximately 45% of the total CES cases. Other etiologies associated with acute CES include malignancies, trauma, infection, stenosis, hematomas, vascular entities, and iatrogenic causes. CES is reported as a complication in 0.2% to 1.2% of all lumbar spine operations. Using data from the National Hospital Discharge Survey, a study by Karduan and colleagues found the rate of postoperative CES to be approximately 5 cases per 1000 surgeries.[3] It is important to note that while acute CES most commonly presents within the first 24 hours after spinal surgery, there have been documented cases occurring as late as 7 days postoperatively.[5] A study by Dimopoulous and

---

The authors have no pertinent disclosures or conflicts of interest related to this study.
[a] Atrium Health Department of Orthopaedic Surgery, 1000 Blythe Boulevard, Charlotte, NC 28203, USA; [b] Campbell Clinic Orthopaedics, Memphis, TN, USA; [c] OrthoCarolina Spine Center, 2001 Randolph Road, Charlotte, NC 28207, USA
* Corresponding author.
E-mail address: Landon.Bulloch@atriumhealth.org
Twitter: @BullochLandonMD (L.B.)

Orthop Clin N Am 53 (2022) 247–254
https://doi.org/10.1016/j.ocl.2021.11.010
0030-5898/22/Published by Elsevier Inc.

colleagues reported two cases of CES that developed among 1072 patients undergoing lumbar microdiscectomy over a 3-year period. In both patients, the surgery was performed at a more proximal level - L2/3 and L3/4. During both cases, somatosensory evoked potentials used for neuromonitoring during the case were noted to be decreased intraoperatively. The first patient had signs and symptoms of CES immediately from waking in the postanesthesia recovery unit, while the other patient did not develop systems for approximately 90 minutes after surgery was complete.[6] McLaren and Bailey reported six cases of postoperative CES following lumbar microdiscectomy. Five patients were reported to be symptomatic within minutes of awakening from anesthesia in the recovery room, whereas the sixth patient did not report development of symptoms until postoperative day four.[7]

PATHOPHYSIOLOGY

In adults, the spinal cord terminates most commonly at the level of the L1 vertebral body. The most terminal end of the spinal cord is termed the conus medullaris, which is attached to the coccyx by a thin filamentous structure known as the filum terminale. The conus medullaris contains the cell bodies and dendrites of the L5-S3 nerve roots. The cauda equina is the collection of the L1-S5 peripheral nerve roots within the common dural sac.[8] Compression of these nerve roots results in lower motor neuron symptoms. This occurs secondary to the nerves exiting below the levels of the conus, and these symptoms vary greatly from more proximal cord lesions that produce upper motor neuron symptomatology (Fig. 1).

Classically, patients with CES exhibit varying degrees of lower extremity muscle weakness, sensory disturbance, absence or decreased reflexes, and neurogenic bladder dysfunction. Innervation of the bladder is complex, with contributions from the parasympathetic, sympathetic, and somatic nervous systems. The parasympathetic system innervates the detrusor muscles and the internal sphincter, which promote emptying of the bladder via contraction of the detrusor muscle and relaxation of the internal sphincter. In contrast, the sympathetic system innervates the external sphincter and promotes storage of urine via the pudendal nerve, which arises from the second, third, and fourth sacral nerves.[8]

Disruption in the reflex arcs involved in the parasympathetic and sympathetic nervous systems as discussed are the primary causes of neurogenic bladder dysfunction seen in CES. Lower motor neuron lesions in this region can lead to loss of motor and sensory function to the bladder. Patients cannot sense when the bladder is full, and they cannot voluntary contract to void, resulting in both urinary retention and overflow incontinence.[8]

There is debate in the literature regarding the precise process leading to nerve damage in acute CES. The first theory involves that of direct mechanical compression. The nerve roots of the cauda equina are particularly susceptible to injury because of an inherent lack of protective layers. The protective layer of these nerves is comprised of only 1 layer, the endoneurium. This contrasts with peripheral nerve roots, which have a series of layers including the epineurium, perineurium, and endoneurium. Although the nerves of the cauda equina are surrounded by cerebrospinal fluid in the dural sac, they are left relatively unprotected from acute trauma by disc herniations or other shifts in intradural pressure. Mechanical pressure additionally leads to direct impairment of the nutrition of neural tissues by decreasing the blood flow and the nutrient diffusion capabilities from surrounding spinal fluid.[9]

The next, and most considerable, factor in the development of nerve injury in CES is the ischemic injury. The arterial supply to the spinal cord consists of the anterior spinal artery and the dorsolateral spinal arteries. The individual nerve roots receive their intrinsic blood supply from both distal and proximal radicular arteries. When compression occurs to the surrounding nerve roots, the hypovascularity effect induces the same effects seen in acute compartment syndrome of the limbs. A study performed by Rydevik and colleagues showed that increased intraneural edema after insult to the nerve led to increased intraneural pressure.[10] When intraneural pressure becomes greater than that of the perfusion pressure required for the nerve, irreversible ischemia is induced, along with significant soft tissue damage that can lead to more permanent sensory and motor deficits.

CLINICAL PRESENTATION

Patients with CES often present with varying levels and severities of symptoms including low back pain, groin pain, sciatica, lower extremity weakness, hyporeflexia/areflexia, sensory deficits, perianal or saddle anesthesia, and bowel or bladder dysfunction. Bladder dysfunction is an early and key element in making the diagnosis of CES. Before the development of CES,

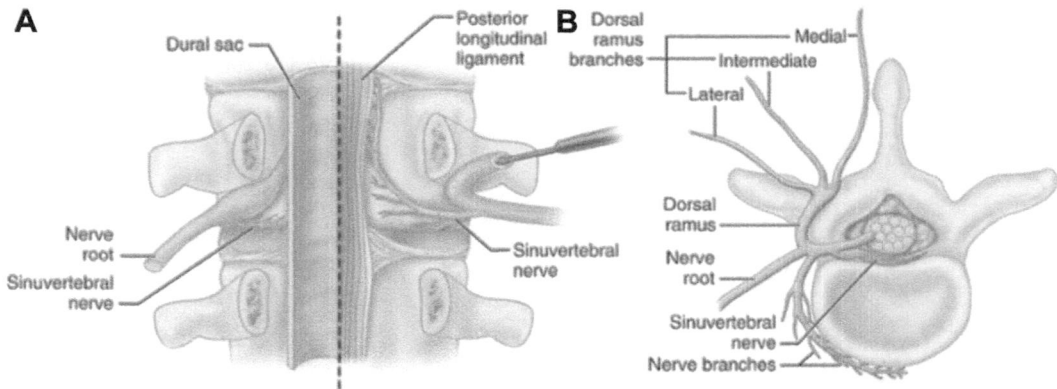

Fig. 1. (A) Coronal view of the lumbar spine with facets and lamina removed. (B) Lumbar vertebrae anatomy.

patients will often describe a prodromal syndrome including low back pain and/or unilateral radicular symptoms (**Fig. 2**).

CES has been noted to present in 2 distinct forms, an acute versus an insidious presentation. A study by Kostuik and colleagues described the acute presentation as the more classic sudden onset of severe lower back pain, sciatica, urinary retention, and saddle anesthesia. The etiology behind the acute group was most commonly lumbar disc herniation that typically occurred in a younger demographic. The insidious cohort was described to present with recurrent, less severe episodes of lumbar back pain, likely occurring over weeks and possibly years usually in an older population. Additionally, he described gradual onset of sciatica and sensory and motor deficits, and bowel and bladder dysfunction. This presentation of symptoms was more commonly seen in the setting of degenerative central lumbar stenosis in contrast to the acute group.[1] This relationship between underlying spinal deformity and increased risk for development of CES has been documented previously and is an important element when considering new diagnosis for patients.

PHYSICAL EXAMINATION

Thorough physical examination of the patient with suspected CES is key to early diagnosis and treatment of the condition. A crucial step of the examination is to adequately examine the sacral nerve roots. Sensation to light touch, along with sensation to pinprick in the perineum, posterior thigh, and perianal region is supplied by the S2-S4 dermatomes. However, patients with early onset CES may have preserved light touch sensation.[11,12] Therefore, a diagnosis can be missed if further evaluation of pinprick

sensation is not assessed. Further, a rectal examination must be performed in this initial evaluation. Decreased rectal tone can be an early but significant finding of CES. Both the anal wink test and the bulbocavernosus reflex are also important neurologic tests that could be indicative of nerve compression.[11] Palpation of the bladder along with measurement of patient's postvoid residual volume via ultrasound evaluation can also help detect urinary retention in the patient with suspected CES. If any of these objective findings are detected on examination, further workup should be initiated by the provider.

DIAGNOSIS OF CAUDA EQUINA SYNDROME

Prompt and accurate diagnosis of CES is vital to both the physicians and the patients in the setting of this emergent condition. Patients who have a history that is suspicious for CES should undergo full neurologic examination along with appropriate imaging studies. The imaging modality of choice is MRI of the lumbar spine with or without intravenous contrast. A study by Todd in 2017 suggested that MRI evaluation of patients with suspected CES should be emergent on presentation, as this can directly delay diagnosis and treatment of this patient population (**Fig. 3**).[13]

A history of previous back pain can contribute to delay of diagnosis, in particular those patients with a more insidious onset of symptoms. A study by Kostuik and colleagues revealed that patients and physicians tend to minimize the onset of these new symptoms. In Kostuik's study, the average time to diagnosis for the acute-onset group was 1.1 days, in contrast to the insidious group, which totaled 3.3 days.[1]

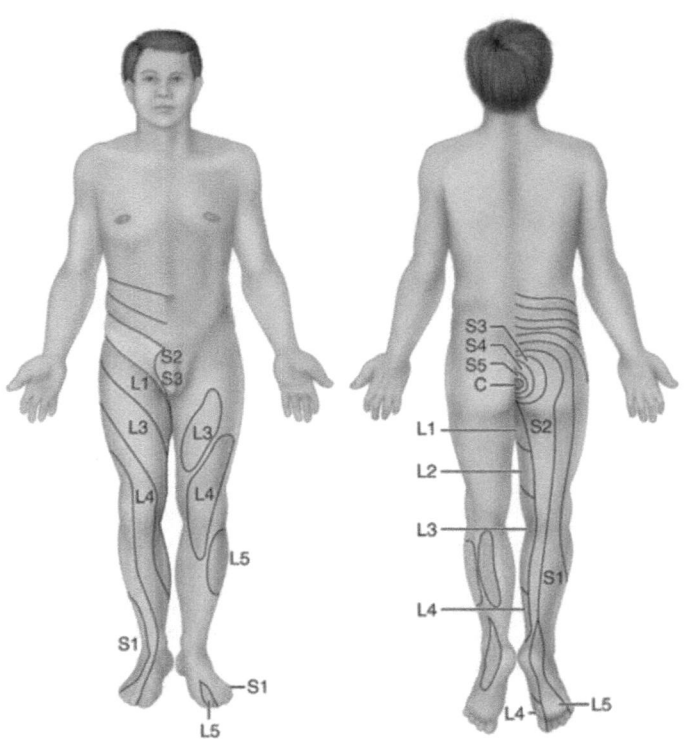

Fig. 2. Illustration of dermatomal distribution. S5, S4, and S3 nerves provide sensory innervation to the rectum, perineum, and inner thigh.

Further, a study by Shapiro stated that the delay in treatment for 24 patients with acute on chronic symptoms was ultimately thought to be patient related in four cases and physician related in 20 cases.[14]

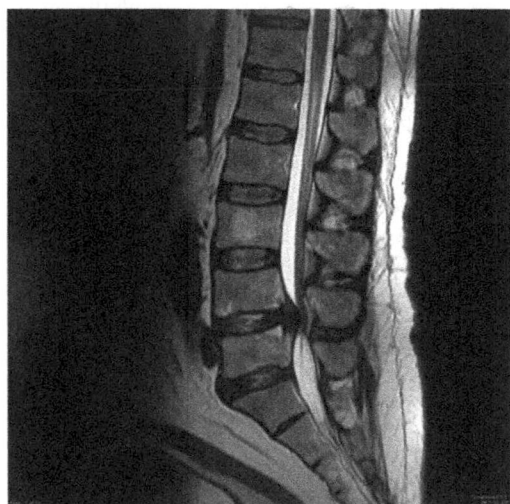

Fig. 3. Sagittal T2 weighted MRI of acute lumbar disc herniation causing acute cauda equina symptoms in a patient.

Additionally, practitioners should have a high index of suspicion for CES in patients who are on anticoagulation therapy. The decision of when to restart chemoprophylaxis should be carefully considered with each patient after undergoing a spinal procedure.

A study by Hah and colleagues states that the rate of venous thromboembolism (VTE) following elective spine surgery is reported between 0.2% and 31%.[15] Currently, the American College of Chest Physicians does not offer recommendations for chemoprophylaxis for patients undergoing an elective spinal procedure. The most recent NASS guidelines recommend initiation of mechanical prophylaxis at the time of surgery, which should continue until the patient is fully ambulatory. Further, this guideline states that chemical prophylaxis is safe to initiate on the day of elective spine surgery. These guidelines are among the first to provide insight on chemoprophylaxis.[16] The most significant complication related to chemoprophylaxis in the spine surgical patient is the risk of epidural hematoma. A study by Cox and colleagues revealed that immediate resumption of postoperative anticoagulation resulted in significant reduction in deep vein thrombosis (DVT) without an increase in morbidity.[17] The risks of postoperative bleeding and subsequent development of CES must be weighed against the risk of patients remaining immobilized and at risk of developing a venous clot.

The British Journal of Neurosurgery attempted to classify patients into 3 categories in regards to severity of symptoms at time of presentation of CES. The first cohort, CESS or cauda equina suspect, presents with bilateral radiculopathy, +/− subjective bladder dysfunction and altered perianal sensation. The next described group is the CES-I, or the CES incomplete, which presents with the same subjective symptoms described previously plus objective signs of CES including hyporeflexia, weakness on examination, and decreased rectal tone. Patients in this group do retain micturition control. The last group, CES-R or cauda equina syndrome complete, are the most classic presenting group with neurogenic bladder and loss control along with other subjective/objective findings described previously.[13,18–20]

In an attempt to establish a more regulated and transparent process to assess and diagnosis CES, Marson and colleagues established a core outcomes set after surveying participants across 14 countries. The 16 symptoms that represent the cauda equina core outcomes set previously were voted on and deemed critically important by health care professionals and patients who participated in the surveys. These outcomes are further categorized into autonomic function, nonautonomic function, and quality of life measures. They include incontinence of urine, urinary retention, sensation of bladder fullness, fecal incontinence, physical ability to have intercourse, perianal sensation, sensation in genitals, leg muscle strength, pain caused by abnormal sensation or nonpainful stimuli, complications, global quality of life, occupational role functioning, social functioning, ability to do daily activities, mobility and walking, and low mood/depression. The core outcome set represents the most important outcomes in regard to CES throughout the world and will help direct research on the subject in the future.[2]

TREATMENT

Multiple studies across varying institutions have investigated the treatment options for CES in regard to modalities along with timing of intervention. Current gold standard for treatment of acute CES is surgical decompression within a 48-hour window of onset of symptoms. A meta-analysis performed by Ahn and colleagues addressed the relationship between timing of decompression and clinical outcomes following CES. This study found that neurologic outcome in patients treated within that initial 48-hour window were significantly improved compared with those decompressed after the 48-hour mark.[21] Additionally, this study revealed no improvements in outcomes if decompressed during that initial 24-hour window in comparison to the 48-hour window. This was also supported by a study performed by Shapiro and colleagues that revealed full neurologic recovery in 13 of his patients who underwent surgical intervention within 48 hours of initial presentation. This is in contrast to three of six patients who would regain bladder continence after decompression greater than 48 hours after diagnosis (Fig. 4).[12]

Additionally, Ahn did not find a difference in outcomes based on surgical technique. Described techniques used included isolated microdiscectomy, isolated laminectomy, and laminectomy combined with fusion procedure. Although no study has investigated the individual approaches described in regards to the amount of tissue damage and manipulation to the cord required for each, a review article by Spector and colleagues recommended that a generous laminectomy might be helpful in the setting of a large compressive lesion inducing CES, comparison with those that might otherwise be performed for an uncomplicated disk herniation.[12]

OUTCOME/PROGNOSTIC INDICATORS

Outcomes following surgical decompression in patients with CES diagnosis have widely varying outcomes. A study by Buchner and Schiltenwolf[22] revealed that 17 of 22 patients undergoing surgical intervention for CES regained complete urinary function. Thirteen of these patients additionally had full motor resolution; 14 had reported full sensory function restoration, and 15 patients regained perianal sensation.[17] Similarly, another study by Shapiro revealed urodynamic studies on patients revealing complete resolution of retention symptoms by six weeks in 9 of 14 patients, whereas the remaining four patients did not have resolution at one year follow-up.[14]

Further studies have emphasized that severity of symptoms on initial presentation is the most significant predictor of recovery outside the timeline of decompression. A study by Qureshi and Sell revealed that the dominant factor in predicting outcomes was the presence of bladder function before surgical intervention. The presence of additional symptoms along with duration of other symptoms did not

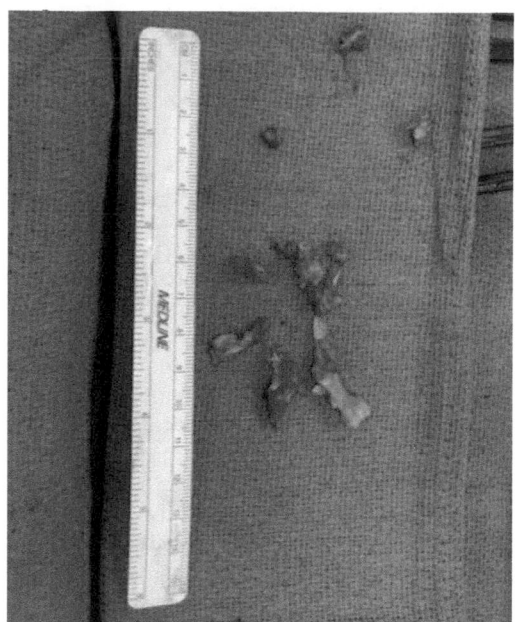

Fig. 4. Example of large amount of disc fragments removed from the spinal canal in a patient undergoing discectomy for acute CES.

correlate with outcomes.[23] In contrast, Kostuik stated that the extent of sensory deficit in the perianal area, partial, complete, unilateral or bilateral, represented the most important prognostic indicator.[1] Additional factors found to be associated with poorer outcomes include chronic back pain, preoperative rectal dysfunction, and increasing age.[21]

As previously discussed, Todd and colleagues introduced the 3 classifications of CES based on the severity of symptoms on initial presentation.[13] This classification scheme is not only important for diagnosis, but for predicting outcomes for these patients. Patients who presented with CES-S were associated with more favorable outcomes. Eighty-five percent of these patients returned to baseline level of no pain, return of bowel/bladder function, and satisfaction with sexual function within 1 year of decompression. CES-I patients returned to socially normal standards of bowel/bladder dysfunction, however had some reported residual reduced sexual satisfaction. Lastly, the CES-R cohort had the least favorable outcomes, with patients often left with permanent motor deficits, bowel/bladder dysfunction, and impaired sexual function.

MEDICO-LEGAL

The topic of CES is one of the most highly litigious and widely debated conditions in spine.

The disproportionally high medico-legal profile associated with CES is associated with inappropriate or inaccurate documentation by providers, lack of timely decompression for patients with compressive lesions, and the lack of obtaining a full and clear consent prior to the procedure. Patients with identified red flag symptoms should promptly be documented and trigger an emergent response from the medical team.[24] Issues have been documented when there are delays in diagnosis of CES and when there is a need for referral to a tertiary center with a spine surgeon and the ability to care for the disorder. It is important to note that although the current standard of care involves surgical decompression within 48 hours of symptom onset, this must factor in for all conditions, including those that will need emergency transport and further workup such as MRI prior to surgery. Lack of accepting centers plus the lack of afterhours MRI availability have been documented in cases of CES delay of care.[18,24]

Additional factors to consider when debating emergent versus urgent surgical intervention are details that are involved with emergent after hours procedures. Crocker and colleagues addressed the issue of these procedures in off hours with an inexperienced staff and the dangers that it potentially presents to patients.[25] The combined effects of balancing this risk of surgery versus delaying surgical decompression for the patient is a cause of debate among the spine community. A study performed by Markham revealed that 62 claims were made in regard to CES in the United Kingdom between 2003 and 2007. Over half of these cases were concluded and damages paid ranging up to 500,000 pounds per settlement. Additionally, approximately half of these claims were made in light of delayed diagnosis/inaccurate diagnosis, while the other 30 claims consisted of concerns of inadequate treatment or postoperative complications.[26,27]

Lastly, the concept of obtaining full consent prior to surgical intervention has been documented as an important factor in regard to litigation risk. Patients should be educated on the natural history of CES. Patient who present with complete neurogenic bladder have significantly worse outcomes regardless of the timing of surgery. However, approximately 75% of all documented CES cases will eventually reach an acceptable form of urologic function.[28] In general, patients must be counseled on both the risks regardless of surgery and the long-term consequences of CES including the possibility of needing catheterization, urologic or gynecologic surgery, or management of sexual dysfunction in their future.

SUMMARY

CES is a rare but devastating condition for patients. It is important to understand the signs and symptoms of CES to allow providers to promptly diagnose and treat CES to improve the outcomes for these patients. Although the exact surgical intervention has not been shown to alter outcomes, timing has been shown to affect outcomes significantly. Decompression within 48 hours of onset of symptoms is the currently accepted gold standard of care for these patients. Additionally, it is important for providers to understand the factors associated with poorer outcomes and counsel patients appropriately regarding expectations. Lastly, further research is needed to continue to improve diagnostic criteria and delineate an appropriate timeline of intervention for these patients to improve overall long-term outcomes.

CLINICS CARE POINTS

- CES is a rare but serious diagnosis that must be quickly recognized by patients and physicians in order to ensure the highest chance of neurologic recovery for the patient.

- Although there is an array of symptoms that can be present with CES, one key element for diagnosis includes a form of bladder dysfunction.

- Thorough history along with prompt physical examination and MRI of the lumbar spine are the necessary elements to obtain when working toward a new cauda equina diagnosis.

- Timing of less than 48 hours from symptoms to decompressive surgery is the gold standard that all clinicians must abide by for optimal recovery.

- Surgical approach is not clinically shown to affect patient outcomes; however, it is imperative to ensure appropriately trained spine surgeons are available.

- Delays in care along with vague symptomatology and inability to appropriately counsel patients on expectations are combined reasons for the highly litigious component of CES.

REFERENCES

1. Kostuik JP, Harrington I, Alexander D, et al. Cauda equina syndrome and lumbar disc hernia- tion. J Bone Joint Surg Am 1986;68:386–91.
2. Srikandarajah N, Noble A, Clark S, et al. Cauda Equina Syndrome Core Outcome Set (CESCOS): An international patient and healthcare professional consensus for research studies. PLoS One 2020;15(1):e0225907.
3. Hoeritzauer I, Wood M, Copley PC, et al. What is the incidence of cauda equina syndrome? A systematic review [published online ahead of print, 2020 Feb 14]. J Neurosurg Spine 2020;1–10. https://doi.org/10.3171/2019.12.SPINE19839.
4. Henriques T, Olerud C,, Petrén-Mallmin M, et al. Cauda equina syndrome as a postoperative complication in five patients operated for lumbar disc herniation. Spine 2001;26:293–7.
5. Schoenecker PL, Cole HO, Herring JA, et al. Cauda equina syndrome after in situ arthro- desis for severe spondylolisthesis at the lumbosacral junction. J Bone Joint Surg Am 1990;72:369–77.
6. Dimopoulos V, Fountas KN, Machi- nis TG, et al. Post-operative cauda equina syndrome in patients undergo- ing single-level microdiscectomy: Report of two cases. Neurosurg Focus 2005;19:E11.
7. McLaren AC, Bailey SI. Cauda equina syndrome: A complication of lumbar discectomy. Clin Orthop Relat Res 1986;204:143–9.
8. McCulloch JA, Transfeldt E. Mac- nab's Backache. 3rd edition. Baltimore: Williams & Wilkins; 1997.
9. Parke WW, Gammell K, Rothman RH. Arterial vascularization of the cauda equina. J Bone Joint Surg Am 1981;63:53–62.
10. Rydevik BL, Myers RR, Powell HC. Pressure increase in the dorsal root ganglia following mechanical com- pression: closed compartment syn- drome in nerve roots. Spine 1989;14:574–6.
11. Siroky MB, Sax DS, Krane RJ. Sacral signal tracing: the electrophysiology of the bulbocavernosus re- flex. J Urol 1979;122:661–4.
12. Spector LR, Madigan L, Rhyne A, et al. Cauda equina syndrome. J Am Acad Orthop Surg 2008; 16(8):471–9.
13. Todd NV. Early cauda equina syndrome (CESE). Br J Neurosurg 2017;31(4):400.
14. Shapiro S. Cauda equina syndrome secondary to lumbar disc herniation. Neurosurgery 1993;32:743–7.
15. Solaru S, Alluri RK, Wang JC, et al. Venous Thromboembolism Prophylaxis in Elective Spine Surgery. Glob Spine J 2021;11(7):1148–55.
16. Li L, Li Z, Huo Y, et al. Time-to-event analyses of lower-limb venous thromboembolism in aged patients undergoing lumbar spine surgery: a retrospective study of 1620 patients. Aging (Albany NY) 2019;11:8701–9.

17. Cox JB, Weaver KJ, Neal DW, et al. Decreased incidence of venous thromboembolism after spine surgery with early multimodal prophylaxis: clinical article. J Neurosurg Spine 2014;21:677–84.

18. Quaile A. Cauda equina syndrome—the questions. Int Orthopaedics (Sicot) 2019;43:957–61.

19. Hussain SA, Gullan RW, Chitnavis BP. Cauda equina syndrome: outcome and implications for management. Br J Neurosurg 2003;17(2):164–7.

20. Kapetanakis S, Chaniotakis C, Kazakos C, et al. Cauda equina syndrome due to lumbar disc herniation: a review of literature. Folia Med (Plovdiv) 2017;59(4):377–86.

21. Ahn UM, Ahn NU, Buchowski JM, et al. Cauda equina syndrome secondary to lumbar disc herniation: a meta- analysis of surgical outcomes. Spine 2000;25:1515–22.

22. Buchner M, Schiltenwolf M. Cauda equina syndrome caused by inter- tebral lumbar disc prolapse: mid-term results of 22 patients and literature re- view. Orthopedics 2002;25:727–31.

23. Qureshi A, Sell P. Cauda equina syndrome treated by surgi- cal decompression: the influence of timing on surgical outcome. Eur Spine J 2007;16: 2143–51.

24. Gardner A, Gardner E, Morley T. Cauda equina syndrome: a review of the current clinical and medico-legal position. Eur Spine J 2011;20(5):690–7.

25. Crocker M, Fraser G, Boyd E, et al. The value of interhospital transfer and emergency MRI for suspected cauda equina syndrome: a 2-year retrospective study. Ann R Coll Surg Engl 2008;90:513–6.

26. Markham DE. Cauda equina syndrome: diagnosis, delay and litigation risk. Curr Orthop 2004;18: 58–62.

27. Fuso FA, Dias AL, Letaif OB, et al. Epidemiological study of cauda equina syndrome. Acta Ortop Bras 2013;21(3):159–62.

28. Gleave JRW, Macfarlane R. Cauda equina syndrome: what is the relationship between timing of surgery and outcome? Br J Neurosurg 2002;16(4): 325–8.

Moving?

Make sure your subscription moves with you!

To notify us of your new address, find your **Clinics Account Number** (located on your mailing label above your name), and contact customer service at:

Email: journalscustomerservice-usa@elsevier.com

800-654-2452 (subscribers in the U.S. & Canada)
314-447-8871 (subscribers outside of the U.S. & Canada)

Fax number: 314-447-8029

Elsevier Health Sciences Division
Subscription Customer Service
3251 Riverport Lane
Maryland Heights, MO 63043

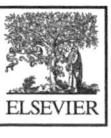

*To ensure uninterrupted delivery of your subscription, please notify us at least 4 weeks in advance of move.